Making History

Bringing Energy Medicine to the VA

Michael Yanuck MD PhD

ISBN: 978-1-946600-32-5

DEDICATION

For Kino, Tom, Bill, Vicki and Sajoy,
who believed in this project and made it a reality.
And for David, who supported its continuation,
so that other Veterans might benefit from this approach…
.
.

Although not always presented in the order they occurred, the events presented here have been recorded and are entirely factual.

Foreword

Dr. Michael Yanuck MD PhD has opened a new door to non-pharmaceutical treatment of addiction and pain relief in a breakthrough technology combining Bioenergy and the ancient Chinese healing practice called Qi Gong. As a physician/scientist Dr. Yanuck is no stranger to history-making research. His work at the National Institutes of Health became the basis for an FDA approved vaccine for cancer.

Yanuck has dedicated his life to helping those in need, serving at rural and urban health centers, including several years treating the Lakota tribe of Native Americans in South Dakota, where he broadened his prospective of spiritual and natural healing. After 35 years of self-practice and healing others, he attained the status of a certified Qi Gong Master.

I was fortunate to meet Dr. Yanuck at the Northern California VA Medical Center in Sacramento where he heads up the center for Homeless Veterans and addiction treatment. Also, I witnessed his new non-pharmaceutical technique to his medical assistant Kino following a tragic accident where he had to undergo emergency brain surgery that removed half of his skull. After a few sessions, Dr. Yanuck was able to restore coordination in Kino's left hand. I watched in amazement as Kino, with one hand, bounced a huge gymnasium sized ball in the air.

While the author admits that this new treatment is not for everyone, this book will be inspiring to those seeking alternative treatment for pain and addiction. I know because I was a volunteer for Dr. Yanuck's breakthrough treatment. I cannot think of anyone more qualified to write about this than Dr. Michael Yanuck.
~Thomas E. Whittingslow, author of "Uncommon Wisdom"

'Healing',
Papa would tell me,
'is not a science,
but the intuitive art
of wooing Nature.'
~ W. H. Auden, The Art of Healing

INTRODUCTION

Little did I know when I applied for the VA's Innovation Accelerator Program that putting forward a proposal for training the VA addiction staff in advanced forms of Qi Gong would yield results that would so far exceed my expectations as to be staggering in their implications.

What follows is the story of how a small, unlikely band of federal employees brought Energy Medicine to the VA for the first time: Our trials and tribulations, working during our off-hours, repeatedly surprising and amazing ourselves, as we labored to usher in this new medical science and final frontier of human physiology – the Energetic Circulation – to the fore; bringing it to the aid of Veterans in crisis and achieving results that were nothing less than stunning.

First were the results obtained with Kino, a former Army medic who worked tirelessly to serve homeless Veterans at the VA. Three years before, I'd watched him fight for his life after a Traumatic Brain Injury nearly cost him his life and only the removal of half his skull keep him from dying. Little did I know at that time that his injury would make it possible to demonstrate what Energy Medicine was capable of.

Next were the benefits obtained by Tom, an elderly Veteran with problems of chronic pain and addiction, who would see a drastic reduction in opioid reliance with Qi Gong treatment, as well as vanquish his opioid dependence, so to bring the project full-circle.

But before going further, permit me to offer some context and background about the project…

CHAPTER ONE

Before the Innovation Accelerator project, or working with Kino or Tom at the VA, or knowing anything about Energy Medicine, I'd been happily engaged in cancer vaccine research at the National Institutes of Health (NIH). Finding a cure for cancer had been a lifelong dream since that disease took the life of my grandfather when I was a child; so that by age 27 I'd performed the experiments to usher in an FDA-approval cancer vaccine. It was the first of its kind (targeting mutations specific to cancer) and launched the new science of Neoantigen Tumor Immunotherapy.

Unfortunately, however, my joy for this achievement was to be short-lived, as I would suffer a leg injury that would leave me debilitated shortly after clinical trials for the vaccine had begun.

Now, as an ardent believer in science and conventional medicine, I thought doctors would take care of the problem instantly. Afterall, it was just a leg injury.

But, to my complete and utter surprise, that didn't happen; instead, days passed into weeks passed into months without improvement; medications left me worse instead of better, with NSAIDs causing gastritis and ulcer, muscle relaxants and benzodiazepines inducing sleep, and narcotics severe nausea.

Numerous tests and imaging studies were performed; some abnormalities were identified, but none that really amounted to anything.

In the end, my doctors told me that I could expect chronic pain for the rest of my life and I wouldn't walk normally again, and I'd just have to get used to it.

But I didn't want that: The constant pain was affecting my work, and I wanted to get back to my studies.

So, I decided to embark on my own course of study to understand my condition, and, at the same time, attempt alternative forms of healing. I tried chiropractic, acupuncture, Alexander Method, message and yoga. Each provided temporary relief, but none ever gave me sustained benefits.

Then, I was pointed in the direction of Dr. Bruce Rind. Under his care my condition improved, and captivated by his skill and intellect, I asked if I could volunteer at his clinic? There, he trained in a technique called "bioenergy."

Bioenergy is an energy healing technique that the comes out of the osteopathic tradition. It's built on the principal that there is a human energy field, and in its normal state it flows in a regular, even pattern. However, when the body sustains trauma, blockages in the energetic circulation develop that can manifest in physical disease. Bioenergy, in turn, corrects those energy imbalances and awakens the body's innate capacity to heal. There's essentially no form of trauma that bioenergy can't attend; and performed with care, it has no harmful side effects or adverse reactions; it gives the body what it needs, when it needs it, at the exact dose required to facilitate healing.

To give you an idea about this approach, I'm going to offer this vignette about my first experience with it: On my first day of volunteering with Dr. Rind, he gave a cursory lecture on concepts in healing, then led me into a darkened exam room in which a female patient sat in obvious distress. Directing the woman to lay on her back on the examination table, Rind moved his hand above her body, then instructed me to do the same.

"Did you feel that?" he asked.

Oddly, I had felt something – like an energetic breeze blowing against my palm.

"What is this?" I asked.

"Bioenergy," he muttered under his breath.

"What's that?" I responded.

"It's the body's way of pinpointing a blockage," he said. "Energy gets stuck at the site of injury; it can't move, so it just collects there. Now feel for what direction it's going."

"How do I do that?" I inquired.

"Let the energy move your hand to whichever direction it wants to go," he instructed.

It moved my hand diagonally across her torso.

"That's right," he affirmed. "It's a stretch injury... Her body got wrenched against a seatbelt strap in an automobile accident. Now it needs to be corrected."

It's safe to say that I was utterly blown away, as a myriad of questions raced through my head: What was the source of this invisible energy? Why did it rise from the surface of the body? What information did it convey about the injury and source of trauma?

In due time I'd come to understand all these things.

But before that, I'd encountered a problem – and for that I needed Qi Gong…

CHAPTER TWO

So, what was the problem with Bioenergy, for which I'd have to seek Qi Gong? It was like this: On occasion I'd be performing bioenergy and finding that with certain patients, I'd experience an uncomfortable feeling, which I'd describe as a funny 'buzz', and felt akin to an aching headache. And usually, when that happened, not only would I be left with this uncomfortable feeling, but I wouldn't be able to help the person, either.

And this 'buzz' wasn't just momentary; it usually stayed with me all day. And between that and the feeling of embarrassment for having not helped the patient, I considered giving up and letting go of anything to do with bioenergy.

But a friend convinced me otherwise.

"I don't think what's happening is anything that your patients are 'doing' to you," she said. "They're not hurting you in any way. I think that when you treat them, it's bringing out wounds buried deep within you. I imagine for the most part they're lying under the surface where you usually can't see or feel them, because you've suppressed them a long time ago. But they're still there, unresolved and waiting for you to come to terms with them."

"I think that these patients who are making you 'feel bad' are just somehow bringing these unresolved wounds to the surface," she continued. "You can't help these patients until you resolve these injuries in you. The 'buzz' that you're feeling is probably your body making you aware of them and giving you a chance to heal them."

But how? I asked, doubtfully.

"I think a form of self-healing might help you," she answered, matter-of-factly. "Maybe you should try Qi Gong?"

"What's that?"

"It's a form of Chinese healing," she responded. "It's a lot like bioenergy, but it's self-healing – like meditation."

"A local Qi Gong group is sponsoring an outreach lecture this weekend," she added. "The Master is flying in from Taiwan. We should go…"

So, off we went to the lecture. There, the Qi Gong master, Master Chou, elaborated on the nature of Qi Gong.

"Qi is the life force," he said. "The Universal Qi runs through all things. Trauma severs our connection with the life force. To restore the Gong, which can be translated as 'function', we have to remedy the source of trauma. This we do through the practice of Qi Gong. By ridding the body of trauma, we eliminate those things that stood in the way of our being fully natural. In this way, Qi Gong restores us to our true selves."

I was curious and asked Master Chou if Qi Gong worked for emotional as well as physical trauma?

"It works for all trauma," he asserted.

And just like that, I was again off to the races: I immediately signed up with the group and was initiated into the practice of Qi Gong…

CHAPTER THREE

Unlike my work with Dr. Rind, my Qi Gong journey was not quite as exciting: The first phase of my Qi Gong training was learning the self-maintenance or self-practice form of Qi Gong. In this phase, rather than an energy healer working on others, you attend the energy imbalances in yourself. This is done by connecting with the Universal Qi, so to forge a direct connection with the 'Universal Blueprint' that theoretically contains the knowledge for healing all things; i.e., it contains the knowledge for how all the parts of the body are meant to optimally function; and by energetically tapping into this Universal Blueprint through the practice of Qi Gong, one can effectively reboot and jump-start the system, so to facilitate the healing.

But despite this requiring a year of practice before I became proficient at it, I was able to ultimately apply this practice, so to overcome my bioenergy difficulties. It happened this way: When I experienced that 'buzz' while performing bioenergy, I stopped what I was doing and performed a Qi Gong self-practice and found that connecting with the Universal Qi took away the 'buzz', so that I could go back and help my patient.

Ultimately, I realized that the reason I experienced that 'buzz' was because I shared a similar energy disturbance as my patient; the difference was whereas theirs was active and acute, mine was chronic and dormant. Nevertheless, even though I wasn't feeling any of the effects of this energy disturbance, I couldn't serve as a conduit for healing to them; I would have to heal myself before I could heal them. And Qi Gong had provided me the way for that healing.

In this way I learned firsthand that the same patients I used to dread were those who had the most to give me – Because by

activating my old wounds, they were catalyzing and facilitating my healing. Indeed, like in Shakespeare's 'A quality of mercy', bioenergy afforded the opportunity to be 'twice blest' – both for the patient and the energy practitioner. So, there I was – Qi Gong had resolved my quandary and provided the answer I was looking for.

But though I thought I was done with Qi Gong, it turned out Qi Gong wasn't done with me, as the group's main instructor, Paul Mok, came to me with a message from the Master.

"Master Chou has chosen you to become an assistant," he told me.

In this way I was selected for learning the very advanced Qi Gong training in the art of Medical Chi Healing.

"Though you have not been practicing Qi Gong for very long," Paul continued, "Master Chou thinks in your heart are all the qualifications to be an assistant."

So, what is Medical Qi Healing? Well, first let's consider what I was previously doing in bioenergy: In brief, bioenergy involves the scanning of the body with ones' hands to locate energy disturbances, and then follow that energy on a path determined by where that energy wants to go - so to release that energy disturbance, and help the body come to terms and reconcile trauma. Well, Medical Qi Healing basically took this practice up a notch.

"Through Qi Gong," Paul told me, "you will become an energy conductor... A deliverer of that energy."

Hence, you could say in Bioenergy I'd been practicing a passive form of energy healing – Just following the energy disturbances and releasing it as the patient's body/mind directed me. Thus, Medical Chi Healing seemed significantly more "active."

And I was wary: I didn't want to direct/"emit" energy at anyone. It sounded too forceful. I wanted to stay with my passive approach and just help others to release their retained energy of trauma and reconcile energy blockages that way.

So, although I trained with the others in Medical Qi Healing, I mostly (and intentionally) stayed on the sidelines where its practical application was concerned and took it no further.

Then, thirty years later, I had an experience that changed all that and led me back to Medical Chi Healing. It began with my friend, Sam...

CHAPTER FOUR

I've written about Sam extensively in other books. So, for this one, I'm going to keep it brief.

Like me, Sam had been an accomplished scientist, who'd risen from bench chemist to Director of a Fortune 500 medical company. Working non-stop, he traveled the globe, developing start-up companies producing cutting edge bio-tech medical technologies all over the world to modernize health care in those countries.

Then, following a 13-hour flight from Asia, he experienced a "snap" in his brain, and, thereafter, found himself becoming increasingly lethargic, unable to think, and falling asleep during meetings.

Seeking medical attention, Sam's doctors diagnosed an abnormality of his brain; in particular, it was found that his hypothalamus and pituitary were not appropriately synthesizing and secreting the neurohormones involved in regulating body temperature, hunger, behaviors, thirst, fatigue, sleep and circadian rhythms.

Advised by his doctors that there was little hope of cure, Sam resigned his position, so to focus on stabilizing what remained of his health. Given the fatigue and lack of energy inherent in his condition, he looked to make the 'best use of self' (so to be able to conserve as much energy as he could) and made a study of biomechanics. He applied this to his hobbies of skiing and skating, and, ultimately, stabilize his condition. In turn, he wondered if he could help others with chronic illnesses by teaching them what he'd learned, and set up a ski school.

And this is how Sam and I met: It happened that when I took the job with the VA, I had also taken up skiing and skating as a means of challenging myself physically, so to continue to recover from my leg injury. Sam introduced himself at the skating rink and we became fast friends, sharing our separate journeys through illness and healing, as we skated and skied.

Then, one weekend while we were skating, Sam confided that he was experiencing a headache. In turn, it got me thinking about that "snap" in his brain that marked the start of his health problems, so I asked if I could help via bioenergy?

As I was working on Sam, I began feeling dizzy and perceived a sensation of energy erupting from the left side of my head, as though I were experiencing some 'splinter of the mind' just behind my ear.

I broke off and performed a Qi Gong self-practice (that effectively remedied a source of head trauma from childhood).

Then, returning to Sam, something unusual happened: Energy went into both of my hands and filled them! Then, more than following the energy path, it was as though something took conscious control of my body and directed my movements (particularly that of my hands) towards Sam!

Long story short, I'd entered an intense 'Qi Gong state', in which my hands were taken to both sides of his head, and then stopped within inches of contact.

"Feels like I can feel all of the static electricity at my head," Sam said. "Coming from your hands."

Indeed, I felt it, too. It was like energy were moving from my hands to his head.

"I'm feeling all of these pulsations," he continued. "And it feels like it's doing something."

This was Qi emission – what I'd avoided for the last thirty years.

"I'm feeling the effects are all over my body," he continued. "All the way down to my legs."

In time, the feeling of energy in my hands dissipated.

"I really felt something happen with this," Sam declared. "The other times the feeling was subtle, but this time it was really definite. I really felt places in my body where they were healing as a result of this - Where I had healing - And the headache is gone."

I stood back stunned: The Qi Gong self-practice had facilitated a connection with the universal chi, so to not only heal me of my chronic, dormant childhood head trauma (so that I could serve as an effective 'channel for healing' for Sam), but also essentially directed me to give Sam healing energy.

Yes, I'd emitted healing energy! Something I'd been afraid of for thirty years! And it wasn't hard or frightening at all. The universal chi

saw that I needed a little push and provided it – so to help me take the next step in my evolution as an energy healer!...

CHAPTER FIVE

After having (as my wife would say) 'gone up a notch' in my abilities as an energy healer, I wanted to help more people with it.

But how to go about that?

As previously indicated, my previous proposals for employing bioenergy to help Veterans had never got beyond the Chief of Staff's desk.

So, I decided to try another tact: I had been seeing advertisements about Qi Gong popping up. Most of it was treated like meditation and breath work, but still it was gaining recognition.

Hence, especially after making this significant leap as a Qi Gong practitioner, I decided I'd put forward my proposals in Energy Medicine in the context of performing Qi Gong.

The VA leadership naturally wanted certification for my performing this practice. I hadn't interacted with Master Chou in nearly thirty years, so I was concerned this might be a significant barrier.

But the stars aligned, and I got in touch with my former Qi Gong Master (now in Taiwan), who remembered me and graciously provided the letter I needed:

This is to certify that Dr. Michael Yanuck trained in True Nature Qi Gong in Washington DC from 1993 to 1997. He was introduced to True Nature Qi Gong at a Qi Gong outreach event in October 1993, where he met Master Michael Chou. Shortly after meeting Master Chou, he was initiated into the practice of Qi Gong (also in October 1993 with Master Chou present). After his Qi Gong initiation, he attended weekly 2 hour-long Qi Gong practices, which he continued for the next four years. Qi Gong practices were led by Mr. Paul Mok

(who served as the DC chapter Qi Gong assistant and instructor), and Mr. Wah Lee was delegated to serve as Dr. Yanuck's Qi Gong mentor. In 1994 Dr. Yanuck was invited by the DC chapter Qi Gong Secretary (Albert) to assist in Qi Gong outreach lectures, meant to introduce Qi Gong to the general public. In May 1994 Dr. Yanuck participated in his first weekend Qi Gong Retreat and met Qi Gong practitioners from all over the country and Taiwan. In October 1994 (one year after his Qi Gong initiation), Dr. Yanuck was judged as having reached a level of tranquility with stable mind-set and not dependent on any drugs or medications (with the exception of vitamins) and maintained a state of gratitude with desire to give back to the community, so to qualify for training under Master Chou as a Qi Gong assistant. Included in that training was the Hochi Support technique. After this training, Dr. Yanuck served as a Qi Gong assistant for the next three years for the local DC True Nature Qi Gong chapter, and also traveled to assist members of other Qi Gong chapters, particularly in Philadelphia. In 1997 Dr. Yanuck left the Washington DC Area, but he has continued to practice Qi Gong.
Michael Chou L. AC, Ph. D.
HoChi Institute Founder and Chairman

Though I was grateful for his support, in the nearly thirty years since I'd trained under Master Chou, my practice had evolved into what amounted to a fusion of Bioenergy and Qi Gong that was best described as BioenerQi...

CHAPTER SIX

I recognized that if BioenerQi was going to gain any level of acceptance within the VA (and conventional medicine, in general), then efforts had to be made to validate it through rigorous research.

The VA Research Department had previously been supportive of my proposals and tried to align me with other scientists. When I proposed a functional MRI study to determine where Qi perception might reside in the brain, the Research Department chairperson expressed interest and told me that she would give me $10,000 to pursue it, and all I had to do was find someone in the VA who did functional MRI to work with in the project. In turn, I reached out to every such person in the Northern California VA doing work in functional MRI to collaborate in the project, citing the chairperson's offer. And every single last one of them told me no. I received comments like, 'Too busy' and 'Not enough bandwidth.' They were all simply to invested in attending their own projects than to collaborate with me. And try as I might, I couldn't give away $10,000 to advance the project. Hence, I wasn't getting anywhere.

So, I gave up. I limited my BioenerQi activities to writing books about my experiences, and took up activities like skating, skiing, singing and dancing.

Then, I saw an announcement about a new 'Innovation Accelerator Program':

The VISN 21 Innovation Accelerator Program seeks innovative concepts, programs, products, and solutions from employees. Check out our application training series to learn more!

It wasn't a research grant, but it did sound like a potential source of support. At the very least, I thought it might offer some legitimacy to my proposals, so that if I received the awarded, others might sign up to work with me.

At the time I still had proposals out for utilizing bioenergy and Qi Gong in the treatment of pain. I'd been wondering about employing Qi Gong in the treatment of addiction, but I thought it was a 'longshot.' But where this Innovation Accelerator Program seemed all about 'Hail Mary's', I thought, Why not? What did I have to lose?

So, after the initial review of my application, I was invited to 'pitch' my proposal to the VA Innovation Accelerator Program leadership. It all had the feeling like I was going before a lot of wealthy investors to back my 'new idea.'

As I prepared, I felt doubtful.

"What is Qi Gong?" I expected the reviewers to ask. "What's Qi?"

And then what would I say: "It's this invisible 'vital energy' that's currently beyond our capacity to measure." That will go over like a lead balloon, I thought. I didn't think they'd have a clue, and I'd just be there effectively talking to myself.

Nevertheless, I delivered my pitch.

Among the great challenges of our time is the problem of addiction. In my roles as the NorCal Pain Care Champion and Substance Use Disorder Champion and Homeless Champion, I care for patients with problems of addiction every day.

Now, in general, the problem of addiction stems from addictive substances traumatizing the pleasure centers of the brain. Opioids, Meth, Cocaine, Alcohol all overstimulate these centers, so that the brain winds up recalibrated, such that the normal pleasures of life can't compare, and those afflicted with this condition go through the day feeling effectively numb – because now the only thing that can serve as a source of pleasure is the substance – so to leave them aching for another 'fix'.

"If I had one wish," a patient once confided, "it would be to get back that feeling of innocence I once had."

Qi Gong has the potential to do just that. It's a Chinese healing art that works to release the retained energy of trauma (Qi) and help the body recover optimal 'function' (Gong), so to effectively get the person back to that place of 'innocence', just like my patient with the problem of addiction desired.

In my near thirty years of practicing Qi Gong, I've assisted numerous patients with a host of medical conditions. Now, I want to train interested mental health professionals specializing in addiction in this novel, non-pharmacological approach, especially at Mather and Martinez where MH-Addiction providers have expressed significant interest, and in this way move towards something nationwide.

In summary, I believe I can prep MH providers to potentially apply this approach to help patients with problems of addiction, so to help these patients reset their pleasure centers, overcome the trauma caused by addictive substances, and restore their true nature, thereby giving them back their ability to enjoy the normal pleasures of life and return them to an effective place of 'innocence.'

Thank you...

CHAPTER SEVEN

The weeks passed, and I didn't hear from the Innovation Accelerator Program.

I figured it was another attempt that went nowhere.

Oh, well, I thought. Another swing and a miss. Back to the drawing board.

Then, to my surprise, I did hear from the Innovation Accelerator Program and learned that my proposal had been accepted!

I thought it must have just been some glitch in the approval process, and decided it was because they hadn't had any applicants, so they accepted anyone who applied (I would later learn this was not the case).

Nevertheless, I decided to flex my newfound Innovation Accelerator muscle and notified the Addiction Department. In response, I found that the folks there had been genuine in their interest and were ready to move ahead: Addiction Recovery Treatment Services (ARTS) Nurse Case Manager, Bill, would attend the Qi Gong trainings onsite; and ARTS Director, Dr. K, and ARTS Supervisory Physician, Dr. V (who were both located out-of-state) would attend virtually.

So, I had the providers I would train.

Now, I just needed a volunteer test subject...

CHAPTER EIGHT

Test subject and brother…

All this takes me back to Kino.

As the Director of Homeless Primary Care, I'd worked with Kino on a daily basis. Since his TBI three years ago, I'd been watching him lumber around with neurologic deficits for years. It was painful: Here was a guy who gave his all to help homeless Veterans; then, on a holiday night when he was out on a stroll with his newlywed wife, enjoying the lights of the Capitol, a homeless guy struck him from behind, so to render him forever changed.

"The man punched him I believe in his temple," his wife said, "because he was knocked out before he hit the floor."

Rushed to UC Davis Medical Center, Kino was found to have sustained extensive intracranial injuries, especially bleeding.

He was diagnosed with a subdural hematoma, which typically occurs in response to head trauma and involves a blood vessel bleeding into the space between the skull and the brain (the subdural space). Blood escapes from the vessel, leading to the formation of a clot (hematoma) that places pressure on the brain and damages it.

The bleed and resulting swelling were so extensive that it created a high pressure within the skull, so that parts of Kino's brain were being squeezed across other structures (a process call 'herniation'), such that vital brainstem structures like the respiratory centers were at risk of irreversible damage. Faced with no other alternative, emergency surgery was performed to remove half of Kino's skull (a procedure called a 'hemicraniectomy') in order to take the pressure off his brain, keep it from herniating and save his life.

As soon as we got the news, my wife and I went immediately to the hospital. By the time we got there, Kino was out of surgery and admitted to the Neuro-Intensive Care Unit (NICU). Given concerns for potential life-threatening seizures in response to the brain injury, Kino had been placed in a medically-induced coma. He looked peaceful, though all knew that this was just the eye of the storm.

"The neurosurgeon told me we can't know if he'll ever be the same," his wife said.

As more family members collected in the waiting room, the feeling was grim.

"The guy went to war and came back in good health," his brother said, "and then he's attacked just randomly on the street, so now he's fighting for his life That's the hardest part."

But the 'hard part' was just beginning, as over the ensuing days and weeks and months and years, I'd be treated to a front-row seat from which to watch my friend and coworker face a host of personal and professional adversities, let-downs, betrayals and disappointments, as he attempted to claw his way back from what seemed a shattered life…

CHAPTER NINE

So, why was I so pessimistic about Kino's chances for recovery? I suppose there was a host of reasons. First was the extent of his injury. When Kino finally awoke from his coma, he was densely hemiparetic on his left side; that is, that left side was flaccid. He couldn't move it at all. Indeed, the injury to his brain was so bad, he didn't even recognize his left side (a condition termed 'hemineglect').

His mental state was altered, such that at one point I was stunned to learn that the NICU staff had effectively put Kino in a straight-jacket, imposing the harshest of physical restraints on this person who I regarded as the gentlest of souls.

Though Kino outwardly handled the restraints with grace, as soon as he had the chance, he signed himself out of the hospital.

Then, he was immediately hit with another blow, as shortly after he arrived home, his wife left him for someone else.

"It's just one blow after another for this poor guy," my wife commented. "How much can a person take?"

When Kino finally returned to the VA (about a month after the TBI), I accompanied him to his first Occupational Therapy appointment.

What I observed left me stunned.

The TBI had wreaked havoc on his nervous system: His coordination was off, as he could not touch his nose with his finger; his sensory system was all off, as he could not recognize tactile stimuli with his affected left hand.

"When I started off, I couldn't move this [left] hand," Kino commented of that time. "I couldn't walk and I was limping around on my left foot."

His typing skills had been wiped out, so that he was dependent on transcription systems.

"I couldn't type," he'd recall later. "I had to peck with one hand."

This for a guy who had previously typed at easily 100 words per minute.

I found the evaluation and impact of brain injury so discouraging that I didn't have the heart to go back there with him again.

Subdural hematomas are known for causing permanent damage to the brain. The increased pressured they cause inside the skull is known for killing the delicate brain tissue underneath, and the pressure in Kino's skull had been so intense as to necessitate the removal of half his skull!

But Kino wouldn't give up.

Everyday, on his personal Facebook account, he posted a photo of his made bed, representative of the fact that he'd got up that morning intent on facing the day and whatever work lay ahead of him on his road to recovery…

For about a year, Kino demonstrated neurologic improvement with the aid of Physical Therapy, Occupational Therapy, Speech Therapy, assistance from the TBI Clinic.

Then, his recovery stalled and went static, with his lingering neurologic deficits no longer getting better.

Follow up CT scans performed on Kino confirmed the lasting damage to his brain tissue in the form of a radiographic finding called 'encephalomalacia' that stretched all across the frontal and temporal lobes of the right-side of his brain.

Hence, as Kino now moved about the clinic, his lack of arm swing on the affected left side gave his gait a certain 'lurching' quality that marked him for all to see as permanently affected…

As for me, just as Kino had effectively lost his left hand, it felt like I'd lost my right.

You see, in the six years that Kino and I had worked together, he'd been nothing less than the heart and soul of our Homeless Veterans Program. 'Selfless', 'hard-working', 'giving of himself' – these were terms and phrases that didn't begin to describe Kino's qualities as a health professional; because, in general, I regard them as overused; whereas, with Kino, they were a part of his very substance!

His attention to detail made my work as a physician easy. When the work got tough, there was no one more willing to step up to the plate and rise to the challenge than he was.

On one occasion, a patient showed up and told Kino he was having some stomach upset and asked Kino if he could help him get a refill of his antacid? But Kino recognized that the patient's condition was serious.

"His skin was extremely pale and he was diaphoretic," he said.

The patient admitted to being under the influence of Methamphetamine. As intoxication in any form was an automatic disqualifier for being seen in the clinic, the patient should have been directed elsewhere.

But Kino was concerned that the patient could be at risk for a life-threatening event and insisted I evaluate him.

I agreed with Kino's assessment and advised the patient to let us transfer him to the Emergency Room.

But the patient resisted, insisting that all he'd come for was some Tums.

I felt I had no choice but to accept the patient's refusal.

But Kino persisted, explaining to the patient the risks involved in his condition, until the patient finally accepted transfer.

In the ER, it was found that the patient was experiencing a major heart attack, requiring emergency coronary artery bypass surgery.

After the surgery the patient was transferred to the ward and after a full day's shift, Kino went to visit him – And got there just in time to keep the patient from committing suicide by hanging himself with an electrical cord tied around his neck!

Ultimately, when the patient had recovered from his Meth-induced mental difficulties, he thanked Kino for saving his life – once in the clinic and then in the hospital!

Kino would say of his role as Homeless Primary Care nurse that he didn't work "for the VA", but for the homeless Veterans "at the VA", which made what happened to him (Effectively brought down at the hands of a homeless man) all the more poignant…

Then, the COVID-19 pandemic hit.

I was terrified. You see, following a near-drowning experience in childhood, I'd been left with a very active fear of air hunger.

Furthermore, I had a well-known propensity for contracting every cold and virus I was exposed to.

Hence, I thought it was just a short matter of time before COVID infected me, got into my lungs and brought me down.

I kept what amounted to a living will on my person at all times, indicating that if I should wind up on a respirator, I wanted to be 'snowed' on morphine, rather than face my anxieties about difficulty breathing.

All this in the backdrop of my homeless patients dying like flies and my desk being swamped with death certificates.

But Kino made it his mission to see to it that I was safe.

"No COVID!" he vowed.

He meant it and did everything in his power to protect me, insulate me and shield me from contracting the virus...

All this takes me to the present: Like I said, I needed a volunteer who would serve as 'test subject' for the Innovation Accelerator Qi Gong project; and it happened that Kino had had some exposure to this approach some years before the TBI when it helped him with problems of pain in his knee.

It happened on a day that I had invited Kino to go kayaking on the American River. As we carried the kayak down a slope, I noticed that my usually robust coworker was struggling?

"I got this patellofemoral syndrome," he said. "The Ortho[pedic] doc diagnosed it. He told me it's also called 'runner's knee.' I can walk on it, but I can't run anymore or go down things without pain. As he described it, it's essentially a done deal and there's nothing that you can do about it, except not be hard on it."

Though I'm often hesitant about offering Medical Qi Healing to my medical colleagues, on this occasion, I didn't hesitate.

Kino looked at me surprised, but was willing to try it.

Kino had (to say the least) a good result. Not only was he able to haul the kayaks down a steep slope from then on, but arriving home after our day on the river, he felt the need to further challenge the benefit of Qi Gong treatment by taking an evening run, and finding he had to finally quit out of exhaustion before ever experiencing any pain at his knee.

Later, in a testimonial, Kino wrote about that experience this way:

My name is Kino and I am a United States ARMY Veteran. As the word Veteran suggests, I have been there, done that, and have the T-Shirt.

I am writing today to share my story of how I believe the healing power of something other than a pill. By the way, I am not only a Veteran, I am also a Victim of my youth; I played all the typical sports, hustled around with my M16, aide bag, and ruck sack, and took on many great Physical challenges.

Somewhere along the continuum, I developed a painful impedence to my heart's desire to strive for physical challenges.

The pain I am referring to is the pain in my knees, and most recently my frustration with my neurological and psychological indifference I have with who I was before my Traumatic Brain Injury.

Fortunately, I met this really kind Doctor that considered the pain that I was having, and recommended/offered an 'alternative therapy' called BioEnergy, later described as QiGong, over basically experiencing too much pain to do the things I like to do – to run.

And, well, I was skeptical at first, but hey, I got a cool Doctor friend now, it wouldn't be painful to try, so gave it a shot!

The Doctor friend, is Dr. Michael Yanuck, MD, and well this alternative treatment did not mean to take a pill. At first as it looked, It was some quack doctor stuff, but hey, IT'S REAL! It really worked. It was spontaneous, like on the spot at the Riverbank. Dr. Yanuck, did some energy power stuff like meditate with his eyes a bit, and move his hands over my knee. The experience was a strange phenomena, a feeling of warmth like a massage, and when done, like when I was anticipating pain as I got up, NOPE. No more pain. Additionally, after a second trial of this phenomena, I later discovered that I could run again, PAIN FREE.

Thank you, Dr. Michael Yanuck…

So, when I asked Kino to serve as the initial Veteran participant/test-subject for the Qi Gong project, he whole-heartedly accepted the invitation.

Perhaps a better question is, What was my motivation? That is, why did I ask Kino to serve in this role? Afterall, this wasn't a TBI project – It was supposed to be about employing Qi Gong for the treatment of addiction. Kino didn't have an addiction problem. So, why him?

The answer runs both superficial and deep: First, as indicated, Kino had some familiarity with bioenergy/Qi Gong from past experience.

Second, he worked with me, so I expected that he'd be readily available for Qi Gong training sessions.

And, like the term implies, these were 'training sessions' (not 'healing sessions') for a project that was about teaching Qi Gong to the Addiction staff. And given all the trauma that Kino had been through, I felt sure he'd be a ready source of Qi/energy disturbances for the Addiction trainees to perceive and be able to train on.

In addition, Kino was a VA 'employee', and could be viewed as such (rather than a 'patient'), so expectations of therapeutic benefit could be diminished.

Put simply, Kino serving as Qi Gong test subject in this project was convenient. Indeed, he was literally the person who set up the laptop to record every Qi Gong session. In that way, he was patient, test subject and project coordinator all in one!

But beyond all these cold-minded 'two-for-one' opportunities, there were deeper, more heart-felt reasons for Kino's selection, too: I wanted to spend time with him and help if I could. I owed him like I owed no other human being. Like I said, he'd been my protector, source of inspiration and friend. In truth, I still harbored feelings of guilty about three years ago: Right smack at the time of Kino's TBI in 2018, I'd been tapped to attend matters related to the opioid crisis at a hotbed of the opioid crisis (in Redding, California). I'd been watching the situation there from afar for years, and now something happened, so there was finally a window of opportunity to really make a difference.

As a result, as Kino lay in a hospital bed fighting for his life, I was commuting back-and-forth between Sacramento and Redding.

In my defense, every moment that I wasn't in Redding, I was at Kino's side in the hospital. However, I could have put a pause on that detail assignment to have been there more for Kino, and, looking back, I regard that period as another time in my life when I put professional ambitions ahead of personal relationships, and I regretted that decision.

Other secondary benefits of employing Kino to serve as test subject would make themselves apparent later; I'm going to describe them now, and, hopefully, I'm not going to make this sound like too much of a 'Rube Goldberg' contraption, but here goes: This project was meant to determine if Qi Gong would help for problems of addiction; problems of addiction essentially stem from trauma to the dopaminergic nervous system – Because illegal substances facilitate such an abnormal and extraordinary release of dopamine, so to change the person's dopamine "thermostat." As dopamine is the key neurotransmitter involved in feelings of joy, for the person with problems of addiction, the normal joys of life are significantly dimmed because of this dopamine thermostat 'reset', such that the person is left in a relatively joyless state, and reliant on these illegal substances to provide any sense of joy by stimulating more extraordinary releases of dopamine.

Hence, Qi Gong was meant to address this trauma to the dopaminergic nervous system by releasing the retained energy of

trauma there, so to help put the dopaminergic nervous system back to its homeostatic normal and the person get back to enjoying the normal joys of life without relying on illegal drugs.

So, trauma to the dopaminergic nervous system cause addiction. The dopaminergic nervous system resides in the brain. Kino's residual left-sided deficits were caused by trauma to the brain. If Qi Gong could help with neurologic deficits from TBI, then it might be fair to speculate that Qi Gong could help the brain recover from problems of addiction.

So, there you are: Some fairly reasonable justifications for Kino serving as 'test subject' in the project.

Like I said, though, I really didn't give Kino much hope of getting much out of this. In retrospect, that probably mostly represented a failure of imagination on my part...

CHAPTER TEN

So, why wasn't I expecting Kino to get much out of bioenergy/Qi Gong? Afterall, Kino got a lot more than I expected out of that single, spontaneous Qi Gong session on the river. Why couldn't I conceive it helping his TBI?

Well, in general, I'm someone who needs to see something work before I'll believe it; and I'd never seen someone overcome neurologic deficits with energy healing before.

Truth-be-told, I'd been told by both my Energy Medicine teachers (Dr. Rind and Master Chou) that this form of healing could help with problems of the nervous system: Dr. Rind had described helping a patient regain function for a nerve that had been severed years ago by "jumpstarting" it with bioenergy; and Master Chou once shared a video, in which he'd dramatically help a stroke patient by emitting Qi.

But I'd never worked with a person with neurologic deficits using energy healing. Most of what I'd seen in the thirty years that I'd been doing this was helping those with problems of pain and limitations in joint range of motion (like me!).

Hence, put succinctly, I'd never seen bioenergy/Qi Gong make a difference to someone with neurologic deficits like Kino.

I just figured that Kino would have some significant energy disturbances that could be perceived and used to instruct others in how to work with them (Which, by the way, would turn out to be another wrong assumption, as the subtleness of Kino's energy disturbances would at times challenge even the limits of my energy perception abilities!).

The thing is, though, (unbeknownst to me) Kino would wind up coming to these sessions with ideas of his own as to what he wanted

to achieve in these Qi Gong sessions. And to test the success of achieving those expectations, he'd bring along his own tools and materials to quantify those desired improvements.

Hence, by coming to this project the way he did (with defined objectives with each Qi Gong session), Kino would completely turn the project on its head; instead of it just being about training Addiction staff in Qi Gong, it would become a hundred times more inspiring – as a project in which a patient's goals and dreams were allowed to become the focus – and then, actualized – in an essentially entirely patient-guided Qi Gong treatment program that was completely intrinsic to the patient's wishes, utterly patient-centered and patient-driven, and derived and determined by the aspirations of the patient for the improvements he wished to achieve...

CHAPTER ELEVEN

What follows are the notes from the first Qi Gong training session. I'll try not to make them too 'clinical.' Of note, this and all the other Qi Gong sessions were recorded.

As well as Kino and myself, the others present were Addiction Recovery Treatment Services (ARTS) Nurse Case Manager, "Bill", and ARTS Director, Dr. K, who was observing remotely from out-of-state.

One final comment: I'm going to keep my voice to a minimum here, and focus on mostly what Kino and Bill experience. I do this because I don't want to lose you by going into discourses of what I'm feeling, and instead let you be primarily privy to the experiences of those receiving and being trained in bioenergy/Qi Gong for the first time.

For those of you interested in more of my experience in this area, I refer you to what amounts to my latest reference guide for this healing approach, Bioenergy Therapy.

In the meanwhile, I'm going to share these observations with you in the most simple, clear and concise language that I can, in the hope that that will make it so these sessions can best be followed.

Subject: Qi Gong in the Treatment of TBI - Training 1
Date: Wednesday, January 26, 2022 Minute 0
"Disconnect somewhere..."

As I entered the treatment room, Kino was already describing to Bill his persistent neurologic deficits from the traumatic brain injury.

"There's still numbness," he described indicating his left hand, especially the index and middle fingers.

Then, Kino attempted to touch the fingers of his left hand to his nose.

"And if I close my eyes, can I hit my nose?"

He moved his left hand slowly towards his nose.

"I'm trying pretty hard, and it's like I'm totally guessing," he continued.

He made contact with his right cheek.

"I'm a little bit off," he acknowledged.

Bill responded that it sounded like Kino was talking about having 'spatial-orientation' difficulties on the left side, affecting his ability to sense the location of parts of his body.

"Yeah," Kino responded, touching his nose with the index of his right hand without a hint of difficulty. "Everybody can do that."

"There's just some disconnect," he repeated…

CHAPTER TWELVE

Subject: Subject: Qi Gong in the Treatment of TBI - Training 1
Date: Wednesday, January 26, 2022 Minute 1
Balloon-on-a-string…

Kino next proceeded to bring out a balloon tethered to an elastic string.

"Everyone knows what this is," he began. "This little kid's thing… This you go like this."

With his right hand, he treated the balloon-on-a-string like a speedbag, striking it rhythmically so to keep it in constant motion, accurately sending it to the same place and distance in front to him.

"I can't do that here," he said, indicating his left side. "Not rhythmic."

He attempted it with his left hand. As he had indicated, here he could not develop a rhythm to strike the balloon with any semblance of accurately sending it to the same area; instead, balloon went off in every direction (side-to-side, up-and-down, forward-backwards), slow and off-kilter.

"I can't coordinate it to go straight," he exclaimed. "I can't meet it to do the 'reflex.'"

Then, he said something that I believe would be prophetic where findings in the energy disturbances were concerned.

"I think this problem is … 'reflex'," he asserted. "Reflexes don't make it to the brain. They only go to the level of the plexus and back down, right? So, there's a disconnect somewhere..."

CHAPTER THIRTEEN

Subject: Qi Gong in the Treatment of TBI - Training 1
Date: Wednesday, January 26, 2022 Minute 2
Nunchuks and prior ability to 'fly'…

Next, Kino took out a pair of nunchuks (which had been gifted to him from an uncle).

"With the right hand, everybody knows how to spin a nunchuk," he asserted.

He proceeded to demonstrate normal ability to spin the device "like a helicopter."

"I can even go so far as to get the whole 'figure 8' thing going," he continued.

This required significant wrist-rolling activity for which he had essentially no difficulty with the right hand.

Then, switching to his left hand, he stated, "I could even get this thing to go in the beginning."

Attempting to spin the nunchuks with his left hand, his ability was significantly compromised, slow, labored and uncoordinated.

"I have to move my whole arm to get it to go," he said. "Where with [the right hand], it's just a flick of the wrist."

"And I know I'm right hand dominant," he added. "But as a kid, I could totally fly…"

CHAPTER FOURTEEN

Subject: Qi Gong in the Treatment of TBI - Training 1
Date: Wednesday, January 26, 2022 Minute 6
Qi Tangibility Exercise.

Kino having shared some of the sequelae of the neurologic deficits from the TBI ("Now, I have a traumatic brain injury and prosthetic skull and the damage I contracted, as I understand it, everything is contralateral, so it affects the left side…"), I next went to introduce the 'Qi Tangibility Exercise.'

Quick explanation for this: Early in my bioenergy training it was discovered that I possess a couple discrete points (at my hand and forearm) that are constantly emitting energy, such that someone moving a hand some six inches above these points produces a feeling of energy that can be perceived. Most experience this as points of heat; others have described it feeling like static electricity, coolness, a throbbing sensation, puffs of air, a breeze, or feeling of buoyancy, density or magnetic attraction. The point of the Qi Tangibility Exercise is to make the Qi tangible to the patient, so to have a feeling and better understanding of the bioenergy/Qi Gong treatment (More about that in the next section).

I do this before performing bioenergy/Qi Gong with everyone, so naturally Kino had done this with me before.

Performing the Tangibility Exercise now, Kino indicated that he was able to perceive a point of energy over my palm.

"It's not a warm sensation, like it was," he stated. "But it's sort of like that rubber ball there, and I just want to touch it."

"Now, there's the warmth and the energy there in the palm," he added, "wanting me to shake hands, like there's an energy here."

Hence, Kino's perception of Qi in the Tangibility Exercise took the form of heat, as well as definite defined borders of energy that possessed a certain magnetic quality.

In retrospect, I wonder about the magnetism he felt? Was this a manifestation of attraction, as though his system was informing him that this form of healing was something good for him? He talked about feeling like it was moving him to "shake hands." Again, was this because his system was telling him that he could he could trust that this form of healing was meant to help him, the way that a gesture like shaking hands is meant to signify?

As Kino himself noted in his testimonial, he'd significant apprehensions about this form of healing, referring to is as "Quack doctor shit." However, I wonder that, internally, the energy conveying something else to Kino?...

CHAPTER FIFTEEN

Subject: Qi Gong in the Treatment of TBI - Training 1
Date: Wednesday, January 26, 2022 Minute 10

Next, it was time for Qi Gong treatment. I explained that this would be performed by 'scanning' Kino's body for energy imbalances. I would do this with my hands, effectively using them like 'antennae' meant for detecting energy disturbances. These energy disturbances usually represent retained energy of trauma that need to be released, so to help the body recover function (Gong). This retained energy of trauma might be related to the traumatic brain injury, such that it was my hope that the Qi Gong treatment might facilitate greater physical ability and function for Kino.

Kino expressed understanding, and I began the Qi Gong treatment.

Now, I was going to perform these energy scans really quick, because I just wanted to identify them without treating them – This because I wanted to give Bill a chance of perceiving them first.

However, following a very brief scan, I knew I was in trouble: There were multiple energy disturbances present (at the left-side around Kino's head, neck and shoulder), however, these were not strong vectors of energy, so to be less than ideal for Qi Gong training purposes.

This was unexpected: I'd chosen Kino because I was thinking that I was going to find strong vectors of energy, so to make his a good 'test subject' for some like Bill to learn.

In retrospect, my faulty assumption and the present subtle energy situation would make sense: First, I was probably remembering my experience working on Kino's knee when I was thinking he'd make a good test subject. His difficulty there was no doubt the sequalae of direct trauma, so to promote a significant energy disturbance that was readily perceived. This, in turn, the exact opposite when it came to the left side of Kino's nervous system; that is, despite the neurologic deficits seen on his left side, that wasn't the side that (as one would say) 'took the hit.' That happened for the right side – where Kino was struck in the head! The problems at Kino's left side were, hence, downstream elements of the primary lesion (brain trauma) on his right. Hence, it followed that the energy disturbance on that side were going to be subtle!

Nevertheless, in that moment, I immediately realized this was not going to go as planned: Rather than obvious energy disturbances, I was going to be asking Bill to attempt to locate very subtle ones. That was no way to treat someone who was brand new to this. How was I going to contend with that?

Then, it occurred to me that, in general, I considered the energy radiating from my palm and forearm (that I used for the Qi Tangibility Exercise) to be less than a typical energy disturbance from a patient.

With that in mind, I decided I'd offer to perform the Tangibility Exercise with Bill, so to get him acclimated to more subtle energy points before he attempted to energetically scan Kino.

In turn, Bill was able to perceive the energy points at my palm and forearm, perceiving both in the form of discrete focuses of heat.

Next, I invited Bill to attempt to perceive energy disturbances over Kino.

Scanning over Kino, Bill perceived significant areas of energy posterior to the left side of Kino's head and left shoulder.

Next, I determined the directionality for the energy disturbances coming from Kino and invited Bill to see what he found? In this, Bill was not able to appreciate a directional movement for the energy disturbances. Given the subtle nature of the energy disturbances coming from Kino, this should not have been unexpected (and, of note, Bill would become adept at determining directionality with time and practice).

Next, I performed a release of the retained energy of trauma at the energy disturbances that had been located. Afterwards, I invited Bill to come back and determine if there was a difference. In turn, Bill described a significant difference.

"This one up here," he said, indicating the top of Kino's head, "it's still warm, but the bottom one [Indicating Kino's left shoulder] has cooled off."

And with that, we were off to the races – Bill able to perceive essentially that I did.

At the same time, Kino was having 'energy experiences', too.

"I felt your presence over my left shoulder," he said, "but then you spoke and you were over here [He indicated in front of him]."

Kino laughed, but it's likely he thought this was because he was perceiving the residual energy connection between us there...

CHAPTER SIXTEEN

Subject: Qi Gong in the Treatment of TBI - Training 1
Date: Wednesday, January 26, 2022 Minute 21

Today we have access to two other levels of perception, thanks to modern physics and modern astronomy. If we term our ordinary sense-perception the macro-level, there is below it the sub-atomic or micro-level, and above it the cosmic or mega-level. The mega level of astrophysics is partly perceivable through our telescopes and partly through our mental processes. The micro-level is less perceptible to our senses...
~ Paulos Mar Gregorios, Healing – A Holistic Approach

Within minutes of initiating Qi Medical Healing, Kino was describing tangible feelings of interacting with the Qi, as Bill and I worked with him. Indeed, he was finding the 'energy experiences' between Bill and me so distinct, so to compare and contrast differences the energy interactions between Bill and me.

"I felt like I was standing next to a wall," he said of working with me. "There was a solidness here [Indicating his left side]. It sort of like made my head want to go this way [He indicated to the right]. And when Bill did this energy effect, I felt like he was practically, somehow, with an energy, pulling my neck back and straightening out my head..."

"The second time," Kino continued, describing his next interaction with Bill, "I felt like he was pushing my head to the right, and pulling my body to the left. And then you [Dr. Yanuck] came around and I felt the warmth, and then you straightened me out..."

"The next time I felt a discomfort at this band at my scalp," Kino said of the third interaction with Bill. "I felt that pulled my left eye towards the sinus area. And then as you approached… I felt the warmth come and my head straighten out, but I don't feel the discomfort growing at my orbit here…"

It seemed there was a pattern whereby Bill was working on energy disturbances and triggering a physical response that was perceived by Kino, that would then be ameliorated by work with me.

"It's like we complement each other," Bill would comment later of he and my work with Kino...

Finally, as I worked on an energy disturbance at Kino's crown chakra, he commented, "I felt like, 'I need to sit up straighter.' Like I didn't want to just slouch here like a slug. And then it felt like I was centered… It didn't take an exertion. It felt more like it just happened…"

CHAPTER SEVENTEEN

Subject: Qi Gong in the Treatment of TBI - Training 1
Date: Wednesday, January 26, 2022 Minute 48
Moment of Truth...

All of a sudden, a feeling washed over me, such that I felt energetically disconnected from Kino and stopped feeling the energy in my hands and head. It was like an energetic curtain came down, signaling the completion of the Qi Gong treatment.

As such, I asked Kino if he felt ready to re-attempt the bouncing balloon and nunchuks to determine if he'd received any benefit from the session?

"I don't know if I feel better," he responded. "I just experienced some warmth, weird feelings of support and posture, and slipping-sliding below."

Nevertheless, he indicated a willingness to attempt the activities for objective measure that he'd brought with him today.

"We'll go with the heavy hitter stuff first," he said, taking the bouncing balloon. "First with a good side."

With his right hand he displayed his previous excellent coordination, meeting balloon, strike-after-strike.

"Now, let's try the bad side," he said, switching to his left.

And lo and behold, he demonstrated much improved coordination with the left that was demonstrably better than at the beginning of the session. Whereas before when Kino tried to make contact with the balloon, it was going all over the place (up, down, sideways, with strikes that appeared uncoordinated), now he was delivering blows with the kind of rhythm that a boxer strikes a speed bag – with pinpoint accuracy, so that each punch sent the balloon the same distance, the same direction and the same place.

"There is something," he said, stunned. "I don't know."

He sat speechless and dumbstruck.

Bill had left, but Dr. K was still observing virtually.

"That's amazing!" she exclaimed. "I saw that!"

Next, Kino attempted the nunchuks. With his right hand, he again spun them without difficulty. Then, with the left, there was noticeable improved, as he spun them with greater speed and authority.

"That's better," he acknowledged. "This one [left] takes more energy, but that's an improvement, still."

He even performed figure 8's with the nunchuk using his left hand.

Taking the bouncing balloon again, he wheeled it with the same improvement, as though having performed this a second time to convince himself it indeed was better.

He looked at me, surprised.

"I don't know what you're doing," he said.

He shrugged and shook his head.

"That's better," he conceded.

"That was amazing," Dr. K commented. "Thank you for allowing me to be a witness to the whole process and hearing your stories. Thank you so much."

"Right on," Kino replied. "Hopefully this will help not just me..."

CHAPTER EIGHTEEN

Thus, in the course of less than an hour, the glass ceiling that had contained Energy Medicine (as well as an understanding and utilization of the energetic circulation of the body for purposes of healing) had been shattered within the VA for the first time! The training session marked the first time in VA history that not only was a training in Medical Qi Gong performed, but also demonstrable healing observed and recorded.

Overjoyed, I shared the recording of the session with VA Section Chiefs in Integrative Medicine across the country, feeling sure they'd respond with awe and amazement!

Oddly, though, I received not a single response.

Hmmm? I thought. How come they're not responding?

Really, my level of excitement was such that it wasn't for some time that I would fully grasp the Leadership's reserve, reluctance and frank inability to be supportive of these endeavors.

So, a week passed and we were ready to attempt another session.

And when the time of the second planned session came, it didn't matter that I hadn't heard from any of the Integrative Medicine higher-ups – Because what did matter was whether the gains Kino had achieved in the first session were retained and sustained.

They were!… And then Kino made even greater strides...

CHAPTER NINETEEN

Subject: Qi Gong in the Treatment of TBI - 2nd training session
Date: Wednesday, February 2, 2022 Minute 0
Retained and sustained!

The session began with Kino attempting the bouncing balloon.

"That's a lot of effort," he said of using his left upper extremity," but I'm doing good. I'm hitting it. I didn't do this last time."

Indeed, his speed and accuracy was essentially the same as with the right hand. Hence, the improvements from last week's Qi Gong session had been retained and sustained.

"And with the nunchuks," Kino said. "Should I demonstrate with the nunchuks?"

First, he took the nunchuks with his right hand.

"With the right hand," he began, "it's just like a snap. It's so easy. I can do this for twenty-five years and never get fatigue. And never hit by myself or anything. Total control, I can spin it."

"Now, let's see with the left," he said, tentatively.

But within a second of attempting to spin the nunchuks with his left hand, any hint of uncertainty was vanquished, as he spun them nearly as well as he had with the right.

"Oh, gosh!" he said. "Now, I'm totally doing it. No, this is, this is, this is not how it was. It was much harder than this."

He even proceeded to perform figure 8's with the left hand.

"That's just tangible things that I can objectively see differences with my therapy toys," he commented. "I do notice a difference…"

CHAPTER TWENTY

Subject: Qi Gong in the Treatment of TBI - 2nd training session
Date: Wednesday, February 2, 2022 Minute 1
'Fatigue' and restoring one's 'true nature'…

In spite of his obvious gains and improvements, Kino commented that there were significant differences between the two sides; in particular, the fatigue he experienced while performing these activities with the affected left side.

"Yeah, I can do this," he acknowledged. "Well, I get tired. I still have to use the whole muscle to steady the shoulder."

I'd previously noted the tenseness in his left shoulder, which he had also commented on.

"It's a lot of effort for my whole shoulder muscle group," he'd said.

'Fatigue' was common in neurologic injury. As you can imagine, in general, when you have to enlist more and different neurons to attempt to perform activities that used to come naturally to you, it's going to involve an added level of focus, concentration and, indeed, stress, so to be tiresome.

But Qi Gong was about restoring one's 'true nature' to the extent that it was possible, and it was my hope that with continued Qi Gong treatment attempting to release residual retained energy of trauma there would help.

"I don't understand how this is re-organizing my hardwiring up here," Kino said, pointing to his head, "but let's do it…"

CHAPTER TWENTY-ONE

Subject: Qi Gong in the Treatment of TBI - 2nd training session
Date: Wednesday, February 2, 2022 Minute 4
Getting into the flow…

As the Qi Gong treatment commenced, Kino commented that he tried to take an active role in the energy work.

"I have my eyes closed, so I can put my entire concentration," he said.

Bill also made comments akin to getting into a certain mindset.

"I'm trying to find the flow and try to just smooth it out," Bill responded. "If that make sense?"

I asked if this was something he did in his mind?

"I guess you can say whatever feels right," he responded. "Feels like it wants to."

As Bill worked with energy disturbances at Kino's left head, neck and shoulder, Kino shared his experience with the energy.

"There's a magnetic force pulling me," he said. "In the up and back direction from my head. Like you'd gotten my head and pulled me up... And a bit of a growing warmth, increasing toward that pull."

It seemed to me that Bill was just doing extraordinarily well. As previously stated, the energy disturbances from Kino were extremely subtle compared to those coming off the folks with whom I had initially trained…

Once Bill was done, I re-evaluated for energy disturbances. Those at Kino's head had been neutralized, but there was still some residual at the left shoulder.

Inviting Bill back, he described the feeling like a "little of resistance" at the shoulder, as well.

Then, Kino interjected to share more of his experience.

"When you started, I could feel that gravitational pull... And I was trying to resist it a bit to straighten myself back up. I wonder if that's the resistance you felt?"

It did seem that an energy dynamic was being established between us.

"I don't know," Kino continued...

CHAPTER TWENTY-TWO

Subject: Qi Gong in the Treatment of TBI - 2nd training session
Date: Wednesday, February 2, 2022 Minute 17
Avoid physical contact…

Kino made another point here, as well, that I'd like to emphasize. He said, "After you nicked me a couple times, I didn't feel the pull quite as much."

The reason why I raise this point is because physical contact in this approach can be deleterious to both the patient and the practitioner, as it has the potential to take both out of the energy experience.

In general, in this approach the hands are being used to sense the energetic circulation. This is quite different than using them for sensing tactile stimuli. Indeed, the patient is focused on energetic sensations, as well. Hence, going from an energetic sensory experience to a tactile one has the potential to disrupt the Qi Gong treatment.

Thus, physical contact should be avoided while performing this approach, because it has the potential to change and disrupt the focus...

CHAPTER TWENTY-THREE

Subject: Qi Gong in the Treatment of TBI - 2nd training session
Date: Wednesday, February 2, 2022 Minute 36

As we continued to attend multiple layers of retained energy of trauma move (both physical and emotional), Bill inquired with Kino about how he was doing?

"I was just thinking," Kino began. "I'm thinking things all through what you're talking about, Doc. And I'm thinking about the two doctors on the screen [Dr. K and Dr. V attending virtually]. And I know you're mental health [doctors], and I'm just bring this up because I had discussed with Bill before you walked into the room about the emotional damage – my emotional damage – that they [his previous healthcare professionals] didn't fix."

"You didn't hear me," he said, addressing me. "Or maybe you heard it? But I'm fighting with what you see on my finger [He indicated the tattoo of a wedding ring] every day of my life since the accident. And going through my own methods of trying to remove it. And I'm wondering if that's the emotional side you brought in?"

I responded that I had not overheard his conversation with Bill.

"But, nonetheless, you know what I've been through with my ex-wife," he asserted.

I nodded, though I indicated that I was just endeavoring to release retained energy of trauma, so to help the body to heal; I was just following the paths of energy disturbances to where they were taking me without looking to understand them or offer a direct interpretation; I was just practicing an energy healing technique that was completely dependent on his system being amenable to releasing energy imbalances, when and where and as much as it saw fit.

"Okay," he said…

CHAPTER TWENTY-FOUR

Subject: Qi Gong in the Treatment of TBI - 2nd training session
Date: Wednesday, February 2, 2022 Minute 41
Getting at the "part that's jacked up…"

Kino described feeling "very still."

"As if staying erect and upright is back to normal," he commented. "But it's like there is a magnetic pull and my resistance."

I asked if it was typical for him to feel that stillness?

"I have no idea," he responded. "All eyes are on me. Even my eyes are on me."

"If anything," he added, "I'm happy to hear about your dance you were expressing. As I opened my eyes, I could see you were on my right side in the front and I thought for a quick second, 'It's about time you got to that side of my head. That's the part that's jacked up,' but I'm just letting the magic of this happen."

Perceiving some energy on the right side of Kino's head, I invited Bill to scan there.

Bill positioned himself at the source of energy on the right.

"Yeah, even before you touched it," Kino commented, "I felt a warm sensation – like what feel you when you have your hands in your pocket."

"I don't know where his hands are, but at the prosthetic skull, I feel the warmth," Kino continued. "And the prosthetic doesn't ever feel anything there. Whoever feels there skull anyhow? I can feel on my left – I can't feel on my right. But I feel warmth – so it's awakening…"

CHAPTER TWENTY-FIVE

Subject: Qi Gong in the Treatment of TBI - 2nd training session
Date: Wednesday, February 2, 2022 Minute 50
Helping the energy move…

Dr. K had been attentively watching and now asked a question.

"Bill, can I ask," she said. "Are you now moving some of the energy, kind of like Dr Yanuck? As opposed to originally, I think he used the word, like, 'absorbing'?"

"Well, in my mind's eye," he began, "it's like I feel the energy kind of pool right here – as opposed to flow and move. But I'm trying to help it move. Does that make sense?"

"Mm hmm," she responded. "And your approach is different, though, than in the beginning. In the beginning, was it more about identification?

"Yes," Bill responded.

I interjected that it was important not to use force of any kind.

"I want you to take it really, really slowly," I instructed Bill. "Just go with what you feel. don't try to make something happen. I have been doing this for a while. So, like I said, things happen fast with me. But at the beginning stage, it's very, very, very important that you just take your time."

Bill continued working.

"My palms are feeling pretty hot," he commented.

Feeling over the area, I perceived no energy, such that I concluded that Bill had neutralized the strain in the area.

"Makes sense," Bill said.

Subject: Qi Gong in the Treatment of TBI - 2nd training session
Date: Wednesday, February 2, 2022 Minute 54
A Quality of Mercy - 'Twice blest'

Bill felt that he had done enough and commented about the importance of staying grounded.

"We can't let your own energy in there," he said. "Otherwise, we're like energy vampires – we suck it up."

I held that that was not an issue with this approach. It's just all about following the energy. And it was my experience that if you do that and just go where it wants you to go, good things happen.

"It doesn't take anything out of you," I asserted. "For me, it just gives to you. Maybe I shouldn't share this with everybody, but I will… I came out of the last session feeling extraordinarily good in a way that I could perceive. And that was. My whole life, I was hit by that car and I've always felt like I am dragging my left leg around, and just it like a crutch. And I came out of the session last week and I went home and I walked my dog and it was like, 'Oh, it feels like I'm walking on my two legs in a tandem, coordinated fashion. This is great.'"

"And Kino knows this a little bit," I added, "because he's gone skiing with me; and when it comes to taking turns, I can do that fine. But when it comes to going straight with my two legs working together, I wipe out. Because I can't get this left leg to work with the right one when it comes to them doing something together."

Kino nodded.

"But since that last training, there's been a change in me that I really appreciate," I continued. "So, it's really a wonderful modality, because in my opinion not only can you a potentially give so much to the person you're working with, it has a whole lot to give to you - As long as you work with the person. Just take it easy and just follow the energy. That's all you need to do..."

CHAPTER TWENTY-SIX

Subject: Qi Gong in the Treatment of TBI - 2nd training session
Date: Wednesday, February 2, 2022 Minute 57
Putting it all together

I performed a final scan before announcing, "Okay, so I think we're pretty well done this time. How are you doing, Kino?"

"I've just been resting," he responded. "I have not rested the whole day. This is better than a lunch."

I asked if he felt up to re-attempting the nunchuks and punching balloon?

"Yeah, I can demonstrate and try," he responded. "I'm not going to go home and try."

He took the bouncing balloon.

"Silly of me to think," he commented, "but it's like, 'This kid is playing with his toys.'"

I, however, held that what we were witnessing was no child's play.

Attempting the punching balloon, he continued to demonstrate improvement, with much greater rhythmic speed and accuracy of placement.

"Before it used to be all over the place," he said.

He moved to the nunchuks.

"Stand back," he advised, as he took the nunchuks.

With this device, also, he demonstrated greater speed of spinning, as well as his shoulder appeared looser, more steady, with less tension.

"Much easier," he said. "Yeah. Yeah. I don't have to look at it. It's just going."

"The goal is to be able to do it without looking at it," he continued.

He switched over to performing figure 8's.

"Just from the beginning to now, I feel it improved," he said.

This was a major difference. He was much more fluid with his left shoulder! As a lifelong tennis enthusiast, it was like watching someone progress in his groundstroke from being stiff in the shoulder to opening it up and hitting a returned ball with confidence.

"You know, my uncle," Kino began. "He lives in Hawaii. He's like a master with playing with these toys. And he told me it's good for me because it will help me bring balance and grounding and centering, and help me fine tune it, and that's what got me on this idea."

"And now I am," he declared...

CHAPTER TWENTY-SEVEN

Subject: Qi Gong in the Treatment of TBI - 2nd training session
Date: Wednesday, February 2, 2022 Minute 1:00
Thoughts from those in attendance...

"What I notice," Bill commented, "is the first time we did this last week, you weren't able to do it - Pretty much at all. I mean, you could do it, but you couldn't. I mean, piece by piece, you couldn't put it all together.

"And when you came today, you could do it, but you had to use a lot of effort to do it and it wasn't fluid. It was very... Well, you were all tensed up on your left side, [whereas] with the right side, you were all coordinated.

"I notice quite a bit of difference this time, where it seems like it doesn't take as much effort at the end of today as compared to the beginning of today. That's just what it looks like to me when I'm seeing how you're doing it..."

Meanwhile, Kino wasn't done yet; next, he demonstrated his ability to touch his index finger to his nose for his left hand, with no difficulty whatsoever. Rather, he was doing this as naturally as if he never had a spatial orientation difficulty like what he'd displayed a week ago! It was an extraordinary improvement from the first session.

"Last time you were hitting your cheek," Bill noted.

"Yeah, last time I went like over here," Kino acknowledged, touching his cheek instead of his nose...

Dr. K also offered some remarks.

"I was just going to say that was awesome," she said. "I agree that I do think that from last week, it did seem that your dexterity

was a bit more improved. So, I don't know if you're also feeling that, but it seemed a lot better from last week.

"I just wanted to again thank you for allowing us to observe and learn through this process."

"Oh, well, thank you all," Kino said. "I think this is going to go a long way..."

CHAPTER TWENTY-EIGHT

Subject: Qi Gong in the Treatment of TBI - 2nd training session
Date: Wednesday, February 2, 2022 Minute 1:02
Precautions?...

Before disbanding, Kino inquired about the possibility of adverse effects from Qi Gong?

"With pulling out this energy and mixing it around and everything… Is there any chance it could jack me up worse?"

I had not seen negative outcomes with this form of therapy.

"I think we are geared to help each other when it comes to this kind of energy work," I said. "So, no, it's never been my experience that someone has walked away worse as a result of this."

"Because I don't want to like be driving home and have a seizure or something," Kino clarified. "Because it's my brain we're playing with… I feel fine, but I don't want to be driving down the road and the next thing I see is yellow lights everywhere."

I offered to drive him home.

"Do not worry," he responded. "I feel better than earlier..."

CHAPTER TWENTY-NINE

Within the ARTS group, everyone was excited about the improvements that Kino was demonstrating. In response to a summary of the last session, Dr. K offered the following comments:

Thanks for sharing! I am also really blown away by his improvements!
I look forward to learning more and hopefully one day being able to do this with patients 😊 Thanks for being our teacher!

To my surprise, Kino didn't make himself available for what would have been his third week of treatment. Indeed, I was struck by how blasé he seemed about it.

However, in retrospect, perhaps that wasn't bad. Afterall, Kino wasn't participating in anything else, so the Qi Gong sessions were the sole form of treatment he was receiving for his condition. As such, there was no other source of therapy to account for his improvement...

Subject: Qi Gong in the Treatment of TBI – 3rd training session
Date: Wednesday, March 2, 2022 Minute 0
What doesn't kill you...

The 3rd Qi Gong training session of the Innovation Accelerator project began with Kino demonstrating retained improvements in coordination and motor function with his left side using the nunchuks.

"I'd say I'm doing much better," he declared. "On a scale of 0 to 10, before I felt like I was at a three. Now I believe I'm at eight. They are so close."

"I noticed some improvement with the numbness of my fingers," he continued. "Not quite perfect just yet. But, oh my gosh, so much better."

He demonstrated finger to nose coordination.

"Perfect, first time," he said. "It's remembering."

Kino confirmed that the only form of therapy that he was undergoing or practicing was Qi Gong. Furthermore, he hadn't handled the nunchuks since the last session.

"So, I haven't done nothing therapeutic except coming here and working with you and Bill those two times," he affirmed.

Kino expressed excitement for the Qi Gong therapy that he's been receiving.

"I love it and I want more of it," he said.

Kino acknowledged it had been some two years since he had other forms of therapy, which included occupational therapy and Sequential Stimulator. He described the history of his rehabilitation, including what inspired him to use the nunchuks as a measure of progress before and since receiving Qi Gong.

"I hadn't played with nunchuks since [the traumatic brain injury], because I couldn't get the nunchuks to go in a single circle," he said. "And so I knew it was going to be a challenge since three years ago. But I hadn't really taken any step forward in this 'rehabilitation' until you offered. Then, I started looking for, 'What can I do to see an improvement?'… And you and whoever is watching can see, and I can see it that [improvement]. That's why I'm still here."

Kino described putting himself in a relaxed state while the Qi Gong treatment was being performed.

"I treat it like talking and listening," he said. "You can't talk and listen at the same time. So, I'm going to try not to do anything, and let you move the energy in such way is that I don't slide the part over. I'm just going to try to be still and be here."

I asked if our 'checking in' with him interrupted his relax state?

"No, it provides reassurance," he responded. "I appreciate the feedback."

I began the Qi Gong session (Of note, Bill was available to participate, though Dr. K was [as usual] attending virtually). Starting by scanning on his left side, the energy path took me to his right, and then to his left again.

I commented on the subject of performing Qi Gong as a healthcare professional: In general, the last thing that I wanted was to do anything that discredited me, and yet I was most comfortable in my skin was when I performed Qi Gong. Hence, this was extremely tangible to me, despite it being invisible energy.

Next, I shared about how it was that as well as Kino undergoing healing with these sessions, I did. Such that, as well as releasing the retained energy of trauma in him, it seemed that these sessions were helping to release the retained energy of trauma in me.

Then, I offered a rather detailed commentary on the subject of trauma: I started by saying that I couldn't imagine anyone who hadn't experienced significant trauma in their lives. Indeed, I held that trauma was essentially a daily occurrence and studies would say that trauma made us stronger, though it did matter how we reconciled that trauma.

Citing the adage, "What doesn't kill you makes you stronger," I described the experiments of H. J. Ginsberg (1974): It is known that newborn chicks respond to a perceived overwhelming threat by entering a state of immobility. This is called a 'freeze response' and is akin to 'playing possum'; i.e., what an opossum does when it feigns death. Indeed, every animal on the planet manifests a form of this reaction. Why? Because every one time out of ten when a predator is chasing a prey animal, it's doing this outer of instinct instead of hunger. So, at the moment when all seems lost and the predator is about to pounce, the prey animal shifts from the sympathetic nervous system-driven 'fight-or-flight' response to the parasympathetic-driven 'freeze response' in hopes that (the chase over) the predator will leave the prey animal unharmed.

Awakening from the freeze response is a complex process called 'frozen release.' In frozen release, the retained energy of trauma is slowly discharged and dissipated, much the way a dog twitches and trembles in sleep.

Ginsberg wanted to know what effect the freeze response and frozen release had on the chicks? Did this process weaken the chicks because it traumatized them? Or did it make them stronger from having undergone this 'exercise'?

So, Ginsberg and his colleagues traumatized a group of chicks (This achieved by cupping the chicks between their hands till the chicks became immobile), then let these chicks undergo frozen release.

Next, Ginsberg performed resiliency testing on the chicks, testing their endurance. What he found was that these traumatized chicks were stronger than chicks that hadn't been traumatized.

But the experiment didn't stop there: Next, Ginsberg and his colleagues traumatized a second group of chicks; but, this time, instead of letting the chicks undergo the frozen release process undisturbed, the scientists repetitively tapped on the animals' breasts. As a result, when this group of chicks underwent resiliency testing, they were found to be the weakest of all – even weaker than the control group of chicks that had not been traumatized.

Hence, retained energy of trauma makes us weaker. It is only by reconciling and releasing the energy of trauma in a healthy fashion that we become stronger.

That's why bioenergy is so important, I declared. Even for traumas that occurred years and years ago, bioenergy can get at the retained energy of trauma and release it, so to make the person stronger.

Indeed, to understand how bioenergy works, really, you have to understand the freeze response and then frozen release: The freeze response essentially amounts to a surge of retained energy of trauma, so to put a person into a suspended state of animation; and frozen release amounts to the letting go of that retained energy of trauma, so that you can functionally use your body again. If you don't go from the freeze response to frozen release, then you get stuck in a dysfunctional state, in which you can't use your body like before (because you're still stuck in that suspended state of animation.

Thus, trauma inadequately reconciled makes sure weak; the retained energy of trauma has to be released in a healthy way and completely, so to facilitate optimal function. That is what Qi Gong aims to do…

CHAPTER THIRTY

Subject: Qi Gong in the Treatment of TBI – 3rd training session
Date: Wednesday, March 2, 2022 Minute 28
"Misery loves company, and trauma does, too..."

After having completed my 'Ginsberg' discourse, I inquired with Kino how he was doing?

"I got really comfortable," he said. "When you started, as you move to the right side, I know you didn't put your hand over my ear, but I felt the pressure ...Well, I felt a change in pressure."

Kino continued that he did not feel that when I was on his left side.

"As you're talking about Freud cupping the chicken, it felt like I was going to church and hitting my own bell," he said. "I want to know the survival of the fittest. Because I worry whether or not I can take a punch? It's not like I'm going to go get in a fight. It's not like what happened in this case. But do I need to watch myself like paranoia-PTSD, looking over my shoulder? Now, I just want to know that I can respond and react like a reflex. Can I take the pressure of a fist to this prosthetic skull? Maybe this is in a way helping me heal to a stronger level, so that I shouldn't have to worry about it?

"So that's what I started to think and daydream. As you were saying about how if something doesn't kill you makes you stronger, I was thinking, 'Well, misery loves company, and trauma does, too.' And I think what you're doing as you're doing that is relaxing me, by making this very strange state of change and sound - change in pressure at my right ear."

"There is some PTSD that runs through me all the time," he continued. "I worry. I got my pocket-knife. I got a taser gun. And I got real guns, too.

"I'm at a disability. I don't know that I can get in a fistfight and protect myself. I do have my daily carry bag of tricks to protect myself. There's PTSD involved in that. Yeah, it affects my everyday thinking..."

CHAPTER THIRTY-ONE

Subject: Qi Gong in the Treatment of TBI – 3rd training session
Date: Wednesday, March 2, 2022 Minute 31
Qi Gong and Resilience

I asked him how he felt about living in the world, as well as going out?

"It's taken away from my sense of safety," he responded. "I thought I could just freely walk anywhere, everywhere. Talk with anybody about anything at any moment. I saw someone walking by me and it sparked my interest and I wanted to start a conversation, I thought I could with a stranger. But now I'm more closed."

"I'm imbalanced," he continued. "I feel like any 'crazy' could take advantage of me when they want to. So, I'm trying to come back stronger.

"The resilience I knew," he continued. "Well, I'm sitting here like a model student, commenting about how much I've overcome the trouble that I've had, but I think there's more to go. I have to be better than what I was…"

I talked about my injury: how it was that when I was young, I was struck by a car, and afterwards I couldn't do a lot of things that the other boys my age could do. I couldn't run in a straight line. I couldn't skate anymore.

But, now, here I was in my older years, better able to use my body then I could when I was younger. Indeed, the more that I challenged myself, the better I got at things. Every time that I go skating, I become better at skating. It's the same with skiing. Because with my present ability to tap into the energetic circulation, I can heal those traumas that my body had not been able to heal

before. And the more I challenge myself, the more I find those retained areas of trauma, so that my body can go after them and successfully heal them. This is the result of the techniques that I've learned in energy healing. They are able to get at the old traumas that are retained in my body and healed them.

In this way, a central feature of this form of healing is how it contributes to resilience…

CHAPTER THIRTY-TWO

Subject: Qi Gong in the Treatment of TBI – 3rd training session
Date: Wednesday, March 2, 2022 Minute 38
From 'quack doctor shit' to building a bridge…

I asked Kino how he feels about challenging himself and working to overcome trauma? Kino described a natural inclination to take on the biggest challenge earlier in life, but that he was playing it safer now. He said it was like being a heat casualty, such that once that happens, one was no longer able to take on that challenge. In this way he described the TBI as having created a situation where he'd 'learned his boundaries.'

Noting that I was performing this energy work with my eyes closed. I was doing this more as something of a practical manner, so to be more in touch with the energy and less focused on anything else.

I commented about how I'd interacted with native healers while serving native peoples on the Indian Reservations of the Northern Plains, and shared this approach with them. It turned out that they were familiar with this approach, though one difference that they commented on was my comfort with doing this work with my eyes open, whereas they performed energy work with eyes closed, and regarded it as rather taboo to perform it with eyes open.

Of note, Kino has shared that he is part Native American, likely Apache...

I inquired with Kino whether he thought this work was for everyone? Or if it was somehow more likely to work for a certain personality type like himself?

"You helping me with my knee, I had a taste of it - That it worked," he began. "And so I am a believer in it. But, generically, without you touching me, without you giving me a medicine, I describe it as some 'quack doctor shit'."

"Sorry," he added. "But I'm a believer. I've seen it work, and I see it working, so I think I'm open to it. But I don't know that everybody would be. And I don't know that it would work for everybody.

"So, I don't believe that I am a select one or a select few. I think it's working and I am permitting it to."

I asked if the tangibility exercise was helpful so to bridge the gap and give some feeling for the 'unseen' in this form of healing?

"Yes, because I can feel it," he responded. "And because I can feel it, I can bring it to life.

"Because so many people brush by me, and it's just incidental. But with this, I'm focused on it, and I feel it. And now I can see it. Not visually, but I can see [the results].

"I felt it that day on the river. And you had me do the hand thing, too. But I didn't really care that it was making me tangible. I didn't really get it until I saw you do it again in building 727, and then I thought, 'OK, good, he's connecting with them.' So, yeah, I think it builds a big bridge..."

CHAPTER THIRTY-THREE

Subject: Qi Gong in the Treatment of TBI – 3rd training session
Date: Wednesday, March 2, 2022 Minute 50
Kino's wish…

Checking in with Kino, he described being surprised at being able to feel the energy at the same time that we were communicating between each other.

"As you're walking around moving your arms, I can feel like a weight of water flowing this way," he indicated to the left side of his body. "It's drawing me to whatever you're doing. And I'm not watching where your hands are going, but it's still moving these weird pressure sensations around…"

I asked him if he could imagine how to select for patients who would benefit from this approach? In response, he offered to volunteer his experience with other veterans.

"On so many occasions, the knee pain patient from the other day, the traumatic brain injury patient, I put it in perspective: 'Oh, yeah, Dr. Yanuck, ask Dr. Yanuck about biomedicine/Qi Gong.' But I'm hoping that you're introducing it to them.

"I don't know. I close the door and walk out. But I know that you can, so I am like, 'Oh, yeah, talk to Dr. Yanuck about that.' I tell them in such a way that hopefully they ask about this without me mentioning it."

I confided that I had not shared this approach with other patients: Despite my feeling that this was an approach that could help everyone (because everyone has unreconciled trauma), I wanted to move slowly when it came to making this work available, letting it spread by word of mouth by those who benefited...

CHAPTER THIRTY-FOUR

Subject: Qi Gong in the Treatment of TBI – 3rd training session
Date: Wednesday, March 2, 2022 Hour 1:01
Unlocking the doors to healing...

Checking in with Kino again, he described how it was that over the course of the time and treatment, the energy experiences were becoming less intense.

"Now, it's just a wave of a pressure change out in the distance," he said.

So, the energy experience now are more subtle? I asked.

"Yes, but I don't know if it's better or worse, but having two of you guys… Well, I'm seeing it. And I want to continue to see it.

I agreed, saying that I preferred to do this in groups, as well.

"I believe that all of us have something to give," I said. "Because traumas are individual, and how are you tap into someone, and who that person is, and what they have to offer to unlock that potential door to healing, might be very, very individual."

I thought about how it was that, as much as I take to 'nonlinear' approaches like these, I could be pretty 'square' in my thinking: For example, in general, I go about mostly thinking that there is a difference between doctors. I mean, we all go to medical school; we all learn the same stuff; essentially pass the same exams. Why should there be anything different between doctors?

But time and experience has shown me that there are differences between doctors.

And in this approach, I believe there are at times significant differences between what practitioners are uniquely able to give... Like there could be one Qi Gong practitioner who resonated at just

the right frequency that a patient required - And that could make all the difference in unlocking that patient's doors to healing.

"So, whereas one practitioner might have one key," I concluded, "multiple practitioners might offer more of them…"

Of note, this would bear itself out later when mental health nurse, Nancy, would join us and provide another key piece in unlocking those doors to healing, especially where Kino's PTSD was concerned...

CHAPTER THIRTY-FIVE

Subject: Qi Gong in the Treatment of TBI – 3rd training session
Date: Wednesday, March 2, 2022 Hour 1:05
Questions and exploration...

Despite being cognizant that the session had already gone on for a long time, I kept working with Kino, because I was waiting for his body to tell me that it had had enough. In general, that happened when I perceived an energy shell around the person, so to indicate the person had had enough energy work for the day.

And I still hadn't felt this with Kino. This despite having worked with him now for over an hour.

I described how it was that the energy disturbances coming off of Kino had always been subtle, as opposed to more intense energy vectors that came off others like arrows when I performed this work.

Dr. K asked if this had always been the case with Kino? That is, that the energy perceived off of him had always been subtle in nature?

Yes, I responded. I wondered if that was because there were so many aspects and layers of trauma Kino had experienced? Or, had Kino been through everything to help him physically, with all the rehab he had previously undergone, so that what was left was just these very subtle energy imbalances having to do with things that could not be addressed physically, and could only be addressed energetically? Potentially at the level of the psyche, and that's why these energies were so subtle - because they were in the ether level?

It seemed that, somehow, the jump-starts he needed seem to be somewhere different than what I was used to. I was used to taking care of problems of pain. These problems resided in scar tissue and

muscles and joints, and typically had these very definite, distinct and local energy vectors.

Hence, was it because I was acting at the nervous system that the energy vectors were so subtle? It would seem to make sense that that was the case, because Kino was improving at the level of the nervous system.

In the time that we'd worked with Kino, I could only remember just one time that Bill and I found a really definite energy vector: It was over his left shoulder. In retrospect, I wonder if that didn't have to do with his broken clavicle? And that's why the energy vector was so definite? It was because we had been dealing with a manifestation of physical injury?

Everywhere else, it was subtle because we were working with residual injury from a traumatized nervous system?

So, I didn't have definite answers. So much of this was exploration. We just needed to explore with more patients who suffered from traumatic brain injury, versus physical injury, so to continue to have an idea what we were working with when it came to the different energies being perceiving.

Of note, one of the reasons that I could do this all day with folks was because my body was still so full of retained energy of trauma, so that working with others was helpful to me...

CHAPTER THIRTY-SIX

Subject: Qi Gong in the Treatment of TBI – 3rd training session
Date: Wednesday, March 2, 2022 Hour 1:08
Leaves or roots?...

Checking with Kino, he described being in an unusually relaxed state.

"It says though you've taken away my mojo," he said. "It's a weird relaxed state."

He confirmed that it was different than before, when he was experiencing pressures such that he felt moved back-and-forth.

He affirmed that he felt his body wanted him to stay where he was and continue to undergo the Qi Gong treatment.

I described how it was that I was perceiving energy at a different layer of the energetic circulation – Now even further out from the body (certainly in the ether level).

Kino commented that he felt as though I was performing some "tickling of the cortex."

Elaborating, it seemed Kino was saying that I had backed off from directly treating his brain, which represented the 'root of his illness.'

His comment touched upon a memory of my work with my friend, Sam, some months back: There was a day when I felt like I could do more for him, yet I wasn't for some reason that I didn't understand. As a result, I performed a very intense Qi Gong self-practice while I was listening to the percussionists at the farmer's market.

Afterwards, I went back to Sam, and experienced what I described as my first real Medical Qi Gong experience, in which the universal Chi directed my movements, until my hands were full of energy and on each side of his head, until he reported that he was receiving a lot of energy from me and it had rid him of his headache. In that way, I had directed my energy to heal something. Where I had been directed to heal something, it was no longer just following the energy, but directing energy at someone. It had gone beyond "tickling the cortex," to directing energy.

But as much as I wanted to help Kino, this just wasn't a treatment that I was going to in anyway apply in a forceful manner. I was going to go with the energy the way it directed me to go with it. I was not going to direct the energy in anyway unless the universal Chi took a hold of me, as it did with Sam, and made it so that I was going to direct energy at Kino.

I believe that this work is about giving the body what it needs, when it needs it, where it needs it, at the exact is required. Indeed, the only time I'd ever seen someone not get a good result was when I witnessed an energy healer push his energy on someone. (Though, in retrospect, I recalled in the second session that the energy had taken me on a path away from Kino and then back to him with healing energy to impart.)

I further commented about how it was that in osteopathy it was said that the best manipulation was the one that requires the least force - The one in which you had adjusted the person's body so that it just went into place by itself. That was the best adjustment.

I also described how it was that what I was trying to do here was get to the root of injury was by working with the body to peel back the layers of trauma as the body presented the retained energy of trauma from those experiences. I believe that this gentle approach was the best means of healing him. That it was directing me that way. And a more forceful approach on my behalf would not do him any good. It would be like performing a forceful manipulation, when the soft tissue was still working to pull the joint out of place.

I shared the Chinese Medicine adage, "You can treat the leaves, or you can treat the roots," and added Dr. Rind's corollary, "So you could paint the leaves green, or you could give the plant some water. Which do you think is better?..."

CHAPTER THIRTY-SEVEN

Subject: Qi Gong in the Treatment of TBI – 3rd training session
Date: Wednesday, March 2, 2022 Hour 1:20
Wishful thinking?...

Checking in with Kino again, he indicated that he felt rested.

I said that this was going to be as much Qi Gong as we would perform today and invited him to attempt activities with the nunchuks (As previously stated, the bouncing balloon was not available).

Kino immediately went to using the nunchuks with his left hand. Again there was progress, as his use of the extremity appeared more fluid.

"It's a lot better than ever before," Kino said. "Maybe it's wishful thinking, but it's better than when I started earlier."

He commented about the persistent numbness, which we would work on in future Qi Gong training sessions.

Session concluded at hour 1:25…

CHAPTER THIRTY-EIGHT

Kino to the rescue…

To summarize, in that third session for Kino, there was a lot of talk, but only some improvement in motor function (as seen with the nunchuk activity) and not the marked improvement observed following Qi Gong treatment in the first two sessions.

When I shared these thoughts with my wife, she commented, "Isn't that just like with a lot of the conventional treatments?... The most significant improvements happen with the introduction of the medication or therapy and after that it becomes a matter of fine tuning?"

Perhaps, and it certainly didn't change my resolve and desire to keep working with Kino (to continue to treat and release his layers of retained energy of trauma and follow as he potentially gets better and better, as well as continue to observe if the benefits remain and are sustained); though, at the same time, I was concerned that others would want to start focusing with other test subjects? (After all, this had been billed as a project meant to help Veterans with problems of addiction.)

But, as usual, Kino would surprise us all and propose Qi Gong for the treatment of another aspect of his condition that would expand the frontiers of what this therapy could do even further.

CHAPTER THIRTY-NINE

Subject: Qi Gong in the Treatment of TBI – 4th training session
Date: Wednesday, March 9, 2022 Minute 0
An assembly of equals…

The 4th Qi Gong training session of the Innovation Accelerator project began with the Veteran talking with the Qi Gong trainee about how it was that he did not experience as much in the way of perceived energy from the Qi Gong expert as he felt with the trainee.

"I didn't really feel as much last week as the previous week when you were here," Kino told Bill. "So, maybe there is something about what you're doing for me, as opposed to what doc did?"

In response, we considered a number of different factors of different factors that might be involved in this, including difference in healers, difference in patient needs, how some healers might be better suited and something of holders to the unique 'key' to healing for individuals, etc.

In retrospect, I wonder that the perceived difference might be related to a number of different factors the difference in approach between Bill and me? In general, Bill would keep his hands close to Kino, whereas I would deliberately keep my hands considerably further from him. The reason for this was because, where I was training Bill, I didn't want to neutralize the energy disturbances before Bill had a chance to perceive them (especially as Kino's energy disturbances were already so subtle and difficult to perceive).

Meanwhile, I'm getting rid of the "Qi Gong expert" and "Qi Gong trainee" references, especially as Kino could obviously perceive that Bill was nothing less than a gifted and talented energy healer…

CHAPTER FORTY

Subject: Qi Gong in the Treatment of TBI – 4th training session
Date: Wednesday, March 9, 2022 Minute 5
Awakenings

Even more than continuing Qi Gong to attend his motor difficulties, Kino indicated that what he really wanted was treatment for the problems of sensory loss affecting his left hand.

"Because I've already retained the reflex in the balloon thing," he said.

As such, we mutually decided to make Kino's sensory issues the focus of today's Qi Gong session.

First, I performed a neurologic exam focused on sensory evaluation. In doing so, even for soft touch, Kino described a significant difference in sensation between his two hands.

"Touching here [the right hand] gives me a ticklish sort of thrill," he said, "whereas here [left hand] there's a feeling like there's a piece of plastic laid upon my finger and there's a distance of this same sensation."

In general, the exam showed decreased sensation for light touch, pinprick, and vibration between digits two through five of the left hand compared to the right; his thumb was spared of any sensory loss, and the densest sensory loss found for his middle finger.

"The middle finger, I can't tell really if you're touching me at all," he said. "I feel like there's a touch, but I couldn't tell you what it was."

After the sensory evaluation, I did invite Kino to attempt the bouncing balloon and nunchuks, so to evaluate whether previous gains were retained. Of note, the original bouncing balloon (yellow) had been lost, so a new one was used (red), which proved more difficult to use for the veteran. Nevertheless, the Veteran felt that his improvement was undiminished.

"Retained," he commented of his bouncing balloon ability.

Nunchuk use was performed next, Kino displaying retained improvement. Indeed, Kino (by his own volition) increased the level of difficulty with the nunchuks by performing this activity with his eyes closed.

"When this started, I couldn't even get this thing to turn one single circle," he said. "So, I've come a long way.... With the energy work, it really put it into control. I couldn't get this thing to spin steady before. This is [because of the] energy work."

I inquired if Kino was practicing with the nunchuks at home? He responded that he wasn't (Indeed, the nunchuks had remained in the clinic all week). Nevertheless, Kino felt confident to perform this activity with his eyes closed.

"We're moving forward, so the challenge gets a little bit bigger," he said.

"Definitely an improvement," Bill added.

"That's why I'm coming back!" Kino responded, spiritedly...

CHAPTER FORTY-ONE

Subject: Qi Gong in the Treatment of TBI – 4th training session
Date: Wednesday, March 9, 2022 Minute 22

It is perhaps not wholly correct to say that life is the same as healing. Perhaps we should say that the force that promotes life is the same force which effects healing. In other words, life-force and healing power are akin to each other and have the same source…
~ Paulos Mar Gregorios, Healing – A Holistic Approach

Moving to the Qi Gong treatment phase, I scanned Kino energetically and perceived an energy disturbance over his left arm and invited Bill to scan. Bill confirmed that he also perceived the energy disturbance.

Next, I corrected the energy disturbance by following its path.

"Much cooler," Bill responded after scanning the area again. (Note that Bill natural inclination was to experience Qi in the form of heat, such that the more intense energy disturbances, he described as "hotspots", and treatment led to them feeling "cooler.")

I invited Bill to attempt correct the energy disturbances at Kino's left neck and shoulder. As usual, Bill kept his hands within inches of Kino as he attended the "hotspots."

When Bill was done with this, I went and evaluated the area; though the energy disturbances had been mostly neutralized and corrected, some very subtle energy disturbances remained in the ether level (about a foot or two from Kino's body) and I followed their path. As I went about this, I asked Kino if he had any observations?

"I felt a twitch of a reaction in my hand," he said. "Like something was twitching."

He indicated that this twitching had occurred with both Bill and me.

"I felt a sensation," he continued. "A very light sensation, of like, say, your leg fell asleep when you were sleeping [because] you fell asleep on top of the artery, and then it's coming back to life with a tingly feeling. Similarly, I felt that growing out of my hand, in such a way that it was bubbling up. Not going up my arm, but going this way."

He indicated upwards and outwards.

"It kind of felt like you guys had a gift and were just grabbing a nerve and moving your finger until you got down to the end, and it starts to tingle and wake up."

I asked if he'd ever had these kind of experiences before?

"No," he responded.

"I haven't felt the gravitational pull kind of effect that I would feel before," he added. "Like with Bill when I could sense he was near me from the warmth of his energy. I thought I could relate it directly to his breath that I could feel the heat of his breath, but then at times he would hold his breath, and I would still feel the heat, and so that is a different feeling. But it's a heat sensation without the gravitational pull."

When I asked whether this is been a different kind of session, he responded, "Yes."

By this time, I'd followed the subtle energy approximately 3-4 feet from his body.

"I'm not sure if you're making the same movements of the power energy as you did the first time, doc," Kino commented. "But right now, my left hand is feeling so relaxed."

Although I was feeling a significant amount of energy in my hands (as I would in Qi emission), the energy path was taking me back in the direction of Kino's affected hand.

"I just felt a twitch of my thumb," he said. "I felt that even in my index finger. It even moved."

My hand had been relatively close to his at the time of this occurrence, within a foot of him.

"There is a 'wake up' sensation going on with my thumb right now," he continued. "Moving over to my index finger."

After some considerable discussion, I invited Bill to go back and see what he perceived in the way of energy over Kino.

Bill scanned, then commented, "It feels very smooth now."

"I just felt my middle finger twitch," Kino commented at the same moment. "And then my thumb twitched, and it's like energy just left my hand…"

CHAPTER FORTY-TWO

Subject: Qi Gong in the Treatment of TBI – 4th training session
Date: Wednesday, March 9, 2022 Minute 41
Relaxation

I decided to move to evaluate for energy disturbances at Kino's right side. Though deliberately scanning quickly and superficially (so not to disturb energy vectors before Bill got to evaluate them), I perceived quite a bit of energy, especially on the right side of Kino's cranium, and invited Bill to scan that side of Kino.

Bill scanned Kino's right side energetically, from his head to his hand.

"There are hotspots," Bill commented. "They're not as pronounced as what was on his left hand."

"I do feel one on his [right hand]," he continued. "His hand is a little more pronated, but it kind of feels right there in his fingers."

As Bill and I talked, Kino injected a response to Bill's comments about his hand, saying, "I heard you, Bill, mention about my hand on my right was a little more prone. This is a very comfortable position when my hands are down, and when I start to turn my hand to make it open, I have to use energy to keep it open… I don't know what that says?"

I wondered whether this might be related to some muscle tension and increased muscular tone there and if that would respond to the energy treatment?

After some discussion, I attended the energy disturbance (mainly at Kino's right cranium) and invited Bill to evaluate for changes.

"It all actually feels much, much better," Bill commented. "And I find it interesting that his hand is more supinated now. I don't know if he's doing it consciously?"

Kino opened his eyes and looked down surprised.

"No!" he responded. "It turned while we were talking, but [since] I'm just relaxing."

Then, he laughed as though startled and tickled at the same time. "This is weird to look down at my hand and see something shocking."

About four feet from Kino, I identified an area of energy imbalance coming from Kino's right side and invited Bill to attempt to perceive this subtle energy, well in the ether level. This time Bill was able to identify it and followed it all the way from Kino's right side to his left.

"This is interesting," he said. "This is a lot lighter."

"It's a different flow," he continued. "I guess if you wanted to make the comparison, it's different from when I am a far and from when I'm right on top of it. You feel them both, but they're very different. Which makes sense – 'Ether'."

Of note, this session marked a change and significant advance in Bill's energy perception abilities; he was not only perceiving energy at a greater distance from Kino's body, but also perceiving directionality with the energy disturbances.

Working on Kino again, I was beginning to experience energy emission, such that my hands were full of energy and being directed back to Kino's left side.

Once again, I shared how energy emission was very different from following the energy, because it was as though the energy that I had acquired from Kino had gone through my system, worked itself into a healing form of energy, and now wanted to go back to Kino, so to impart healing energy to him.

I asked Kino if he was experiencing anything right now?

"I'm not really sleepy, but I'm so relaxed," he responded. "I feel hopeful – Maybe it's placebo? – that you've got something to do with that. Again, no gravity-like pulls in any direction at any time during the session today."

It was my experience that Qi emission was accompanied by a feeling of relaxation, although that 'relaxation' was typically more localized (i.e., just where my hand was), and I wondered if this more full-body relaxation was because Kino's primary injury was less localized and more generalized; i.e., it wasn't that he just had some local nerve damage at his hand, but rather this stemmed from an

injury to his brain, which had effects essentially everywhere in his body.

I asked if he'd had this kind of experience of intense relaxation in the previous Qi Gong sessions?

"No," he responded. "I felt relaxed, but now I feel like I might fall asleep."

"I feel really balanced," he continued, his eyes closed. "And the weight of my arms on my thighs feels really equal. Like I don't have to use any effort to keep my hands open. I feel like my right hand is open a little bit more than my left hand. I'm trying not to look - and I haven't looked – but I'd be surprised if my hands were not open, laying on their backs."

Indeed, his hand was open, palms up and 'laying on their backs.'

I commented that performing Chi emission has taken me 30 years achieve and wondered aloud how long it would take Bill to reach that point? Then, I invited Bill to scan over Kino. He scanned both Kino's right and left sides, as well as his front and back.

"It feels smooth pretty much everywhere," he concluded. "He feels centered, even and balanced. I don't feel any frictions anywhere..."

CHAPTER FORTY-THREE

Subject: Qi Gong in the Treatment of TBI – 4th training session
Date: Wednesday, March 9, 2022 Minute 59
Shell effect

At this time Bill intuited that we had done enough and expressed concern that we might push the body too far if we continued.

"I've had the experience where, sometimes, I've made a bunch of progress [with a patient] and then I push it a little bit, and the body like says, 'Well, I was happy where I was'," he commented. "So, I'm a little worried."

I responded that it was my experience that the body could (and would) tell us when it had received enough by effectively "pushing back."

"In general, it puts an energy 'shell' around itself," I said, "so to say, 'I am done… No more for today.'"

Then, as it happened (at that very moment!), I felt the 'shell effect' around Kino, like we had just got there...

CHAPTER FORTY-FOUR

Subject: Qi Gong in the Treatment of TBI – 4th training session
Date: Wednesday, March 9, 2022 Hour 1:00
"More the same than different…"

Though concerned about interrupting (and disrupting) Kino's deep-state of relaxation, I inquired with Kino if it was okay if we re-evaluated his sensation?

"Yes," he said, enthusiastically. "I'm looking at my hands and they look totally rested," Kino commented. "They look like mirrors of each other. The left feels just like the right. I guess your words of balance or whatever. I'm thinking about how I tried to touch my nose with my one finger, and I'm thinking that it's going to be perfect…"

We began with a generalized overall evaluation of light touch between the digits of the two hands: For all the digits of the right hand he described feeling "a distinct touch, but on every single finger of the left, there was a 'tickle' sensation."

We compared the sensation between the individual digits between the two hands. As with the beginning of the session, the sensation between his thumbs felt the same. Then, as I moved to the right and left index fingers, he indicated there was a change.

"It's strange," he said. "They feel the same, but there's an electric feeling there on the left. It's like a shock."

Asked if this represented a change between the beginning of the session, he responded in the affirmative: "Yes, it felt more the same than different."

We went to the middle finger.

"Yes, more the same than different," he responded.

Ring finger.

"Yes, more the same than different," he said for the ring finger. "You did something here."

Pinky fingers.

"Yes, more the same than different," he said for the pinky finger. "You've done something..."

CHAPTER FORTY-FIVE

Subject: Qi Gong in the Treatment of TBI – 4th training session
Date: Wednesday, March 9, 2022 Hour 1:04
Switched off…

Next, we evaluated Kino for pinprick sensation between his two hands.

"So similar," he said of the sensation between his hands now. "There is a change."

Interestingly, he commented that this sensation improved with each successive sharp touch.

"It changed with each jab," he said of the pinprick sensation, "and eventually got prickly after you touched it four times."

Pinprick sensation at the left middle finger he described as "less prickly, though an improvement… It's the most affected even before we started."

Going next to vibration, the pattern of improvement was essentially the same.

"So similar," he said of the sensation between the digits of his two hands. "Very much the same when it comes to vibration."

But his left middle finger again did the worst on testing (This time with vibration), and I was inclined to reattempt Qi Healing.

However, the moment I attempted such, it quickly became apparent that I could do no more.

"There's no charge that I feel right now," I conceded. "This is as much as I feel we can do for you today."

Indeed, I'd experienced no energy sensation at all coming from Kino. It was just as though the energetic circulation had 'switched off'…

CHAPTER FORTY-SIX

Subject: Qi Gong in the Treatment of TBI – 4th training session
Date: Wednesday, March 9, 2022 Hour 1:08

Kino snapped his fingers.

"This was something I couldn't do for the longest time," he said. "Make a similar snap. This one was always sharp and crisp," he said of the right hand. Then, he went to the left. "It still doesn't have that crisp sound, but it sounds very similar."

He attempted a nunchuck and it was much improved – not only for making circles, but also for performing the figure eights.

"This is improving," he said. "It's so much better than the first effort. And it's improving – that's how I'm able to twist the wrist more.... I'm getting a little bit closer to equal."

Next, he went to the bouncing balloon; however, before punching it, he first he attempted balancing the balloon in his hands.

"You see, my sensation of touch, weight and pressure is altered," he said, "so now I got it and I'm focusing on it."

Then, he demonstrated extreme improvement with the bouncing balloon for his left hand, so that it was basically equal to his ability with the right.

Kino let his head fall back and shoulders drop, as he stood, startled, astonished and amazed.

"That's way better," he said. "It's silly, but it's so simple – The way it goes is you need to be able to guess the amount of reflex to have to snap it and hit it back, and it's improved. Where reflex was the biggest barrier, it's gotten a lot better."

He sat, reflecting.

"Way different!" he declared. "I don't even know how to describe it. There was a lot more energy 'pull' last time, but now I just sat here and you guys just relaxed me. And now I'm sitting here with my hands exactly the same..."

CHAPTER FORTY-SEVEN

Subject: Qi Gong in the Treatment of TBI – 4th training session
Date: Wednesday, March 9, 2022 Hour 1:13

Dr. K had arrived late, so I explained what had happened in the course of the session, summarizing what had occurred, saying Kino had sensations of twitching and tingling that he hadn't had in prior sessions; and lo and behold at the end of the session, he did so much better for sensory perception (including light touch, pinprick and vibration) than he had at the beginning of the session.

There were still some significant sensory deficits (especially involving his middle finger), and we'll see if that responds to future Qi Gong sessions.

Meanwhile, his accuracy and dexterity with the nunchuks and the bouncing balloon were better than ever before, and the change between the beginning and end of the session more stunning - Especially with this new bouncing balloon, for which had had significant difficulty at the beginning of the session and at the end performed so well. It was such a demonstrable difference between the beginning and the end...

CHAPTER FORTY-EIGHT

Subject: Qi Gong in the Treatment of TBI – 4th training session
Date: Wednesday, March 9, 2022 Hour 1:16
Typical session?

Dr. K inquired how the training session might be different from how I would perform an individual session with a patient?

"How often in a standard session do you step away?" she asked. "Reassess? Talk to the person? Go back? Is it a continuous flow? Does it depend on the session? When do you figure out how to start and stop?"

I felt my 'standard session' was a continuous flow that depended on the individual.

I continued that there might be less talking and teaching in such a session (so that the patient could focus inwards while performing the Qi Healing).

I commented that the scientist inside of me wanted to remove all conversation from these sessions, so that they could be more energy-based (and the energy interaction) and less of what could be judged "talk therapy."

However, the healer inside of me, wanted to bring in all the factors that I thought would help: the energy work; the interactive conversation with the patient; finding out what the patient was feeling as we went along.

Finally, in answer of Dr. K's question, a typical session ended when either there was no more energy for me to perceive (so to indicate that I could do no more), or else I perceived an energy shell around the patient, so to indicate that the patient had had enough. Both of which happened this time...

CHAPTER FORTY-NINE

Subject: Qi Gong in the Treatment of TBI – 4th training session
Date: Wednesday, March 9, 2022 Hour 1:20

Kino wanted to respond to Dr. K's question by describing his experience with me when performing Qi Gong.

"Previously, when he helped me with my knee, we didn't take any pause for questions and answers or something like that," he said. "It was just some awesome magic that he did, and I didn't really ask any questions afterwards. I just felt better."

Then, he turned to me. "Thank you."

Remembering that experience along the river, I thought I recalled it was a very short "session."

"Yes," he responded. "Maybe 8 to 10 minutes."

That was longer than I remembered. Nevertheless, I commented that these sessions were taking a significant amount of time compared to usual, and these energy disturbances were relatively slow to be corrected, I wondered if this was because a condition like traumatic brain injury was so much more involved than say the condition that has been affecting his knee? That the residual energy disturbances from the traumatic brain injury were more complex and complicated than what there was at his knee?

"And I don't recall you teaching anything," Kino added. "You were just doing it."

"But I'm sitting here," he added, "thinking about the 'layers' and you talking about things being 'subtle', and I'm just sitting here doing this (Rubbing between his fingers) and it's still there (Residual sensory loss) and I'm just wondering if you can give me some

acetylcysteine to make this nerve work right faster? Give me some fake myelin or something?"

It takes time, I responded. There are layers of retained energy of trauma to get through. The injury might have happened overnight, but in my experience, it took time to reconcile trauma.

I mean, look at me: The traumatic experience that led me to Qi Gong occurred over thirty years ago, and I was still working through elements of that trauma. Nevertheless, as long as I saw beneficial progress through the application of Qi Gong on a daily basis, then (no matter how incremental) I was willing to accept that slow and steady process.

However, as opposed to me, it seemed it was Kino's natural inclination to want to hasten that process.

"At this point, I just want to push it farther and farther and farther," Kino responded. "I want to take advantage of you guys for this…"

CHAPTER FIFTY

Subject: Qi Gong in the Treatment of TBI – 4th training session
Date: Wednesday, March 9, 2022 Hour 1:24

Kino raised the question of challenging himself, describing how it was that his brother wanted his right arm to be tied to his side, so that he would have to use the left.

"I wonder if I need to challenge myself like that?" he said. "With everything – With my yard work? With gardening? With writing and typing? Eating?"

I agreed that the more you challenge yourself, the more your body discovers what needs to be healed. It was the way I approached my own recovery from trauma.

I talked about Qi Gong self-practice, and said that that was something I practiced every day, and invited to teach Kino that practice, so that he could do this work on the own. indeed, I was making efforts to teach Bill and Dr. K this self-practice.

"I'll see," Kino responded. "Now, I receive it, but I don't know if I want to be a provider of it. Even if it's for myself, because I'm kind of selfish. I'd like what you guys are doing here."

I responded that I was happy to follow his lead. The last thing I wanted to do with this work was force anything; I wanted to go at his speed and with his intuition - How he thought he could best benefit from this kind of work.

As stated previously, where this work was concerned, I held it gave the body what it needed, where it needed it, when it needed it, at the exact dose required.

Therefore, I would trust his judgment and intuition - what he was feeling - and just go with what his body-mind was telling him.

"You talk about challenging yourself," he commented, "and challenging yourself is a survival of the fittest tactic. Like when you were talking about the chickens."

Yes, challenging yourself and trauma has the potential to make you stronger. Because according to scientific studies like the Ginsberg experiments, trauma satisfactorily reconciled in a healthy fashion leaves you stronger. Now, in the work we're doing here (i.e., releasing the retained energy of trauma), we're looking to apply Qi Gong for this purpose...

CHAPTER FIFTY-ONE

Bringing back life!...

Alright, so in this 4th session with Kino, he'd again demonstrated marked benefits with Qi Gong – this time showcasing improvements for problems of sensory loss that had been present since the time of his traumatic brain injury three years ago!

In the course of the session, he described 'tingling' and 'twitching' sensations in that affected hand (especially in the beginning of the session) suggestive that there were some general 'awakenings' of the nerves of his hand via the energy healing.

As usual, the benefits Kino sustained have well exceeded my expectations. It's like something out of Oliver Sacks' "Awakenings," when he administered L-DOPA to those victims of the 1918 influenza pandemic who were left with advanced Parkinsonism and essentially brought them back to life! Watching Kino progress in these Qi Gong sessions, I has been like that! And this with bioenergy and Qi Gong – working with the energetic circulation of the body. This last frontier of medical science that Traditional Chinese Medicine and native people have been working with for thousands of years, and conventional medicine has in no way caught up with yet, because it has defied our ability to measure. Indeed, when it comes to our present tools, we might as well be the apes scratching at the Monolith from the 2001 – A Space Odyssey – we have no idea what we've found and how to evaluate it.

In truth, at times I wondered if I wasn't in that camp, as well; i.e., that I, too, didn't know what I was dealing with.

But, really, I'd had enough experiences to know that the only outcome with Qi Gong and bioenergy was healing.

Let me share an experience from twenty years ago...

CHAPTER FIFTY-TWO

Fear in energy medicine.

Fear of energy transference is deeply rooted in some forms of energy medicine practice. For example, on meeting Qi Gong master Dr. Chao (a member of President Clinton's Executive Committee on Alternative Medicine), he complained of having a 'kidney problem.' I offered to treat him using bioenergy. He accepted, and afterward, said he felt better, acknowledging my ability for 'moving chi.' But he left me with a warning; cautioning me to be careful; saying that I could be affected by recipients' 'bad energy.'

Speaking plainly, I reject this notion; energy disturbances are not contagions to be quarantined; they are the residual of unresolved trauma to be attended and reconciled. Indeed, it is my experience that healing others through bioenergy only facilitates your own healing, and poses no harm to you.

Only once did I fear 'catching' a recipient's 'bad' energy in a Qi Gong/bioenergy session. It happened while I was working with Brian who suffered from a painful, neurodegenerative condition. Of all the illnesses out there, it's neurological disorders that frighten me most. So, when the path of Brian's energy flowed towards me, the thought of being 'infected' with his condition scared me, and I purposely made an effort to avoid it.

Afterwards, I regretted my conduct during this interaction; when I worked with Brian again and the energy again moved in my direction, I didn't shrink this time. And as our energies merge, I experienced a feeling of being at one with everything around me; time slowed, and nothing seemed to matter outside of helping him; the energy encircled me, and flowed upward, and imparted a deep

feeling of reverence; even after the bioenergy session, its therapeutic effects continued to benefit me.

This has been my pattern for the last thirty years…

CHAPTER FIFTY-THREE

Subject: Qi Gong in the Treatment of TBI – 5th training session
Date: Wednesday, March 16, 2022 Minute 0:00

The 5th Qi Gong training session with Kino began with him describing a problem of pulled muscle affecting his back that he experienced on his way to work.

"I have a pinching pain when I take a deep breath," he said. "It is similar to my pneumothorax pain. When I rub against the wall, it gets better. Right there in the middle of my back."

The pneumothorax happened after his TBI, in a freak accident when he slid on some gravel while he was driving his motorcycle. He broke his left clavicle then, too.

"It's [the pinching feeling] along the trapezius bottom near the spinal center over here," he said, indicating its location at the left upper back.

Kino indicated that efforts at stretching were not helpful, and rather than facilitating relief, it "provoked" more pain.

Then, he put his hands out, suggestive of the way bioenergy/Qi Gong is performed and said, "I don't know if you can fix it?"

Nodding, I thought this might be an opportunity for Bill to experience a distinct energy disturbance vector related to pain, rather than these very subtle ones we'd been working with related to the TBI.

However, first, I wanted to evaluate for the persistence of gains achieved over the past weeks...

CHAPTER FIFTY-FOUR

Subject: Qi Gong in the Treatment of TBI – 5th training session
Date: Wednesday, March 16, 2022 Minute 2

Kino insisted that his improvements in sensation had been retained from the previous Qi Gong session a week ago, with the exception of his left middle finger which continued to be numb, though there was a "shocking" sensation there whenever he made contact with something.

"Like electrical shocks," he said.

He said that he had not had these electrical sensations in his fingers prior to the Qi Gong treatment.

"Before, it was like there was plastic in-between my skin," he said. "Now, the shock is more of a sensation."

Hence, it seemed that the sensation was coming back, and this electrical sensation was a prelude to that.

"That is correct," the veteran affirmed.

In general, the sensory exam confirmed the veteran's assertion of the persistence and retention of improved sensation from the previous Qi Gong treatment has been retained…

CHAPTER FIFTY-FIVE

Subject: Qi Gong in the Treatment of TBI – 5th training session
Date: Wednesday, March 16, 2022 Minute 10
"...super sensitive..."

The veteran also described being more sensitive to the application of electrical stimulation to his left hand, especially as pertained to the use of his sequential stimulation unit.

"I was like, 'Holy moly, get it off'," he said of an attempt to apply sequential stimulation to his left hand. "It was super sensitive to the shock."

He indicated that this was not the case when he applied the sequential stimulation to his left arm; it was just the application of this device to the digits of his left hand that was "unbearable", where this had not been the case before.

Indeed, it seemed to me that the nerves in his hand had gone from 'dead' to quite alive and just waiting to become more fully functional...

CHAPTER FIFTY-SIX

Subject: Qi Gong in the Treatment of TBI – 5th training session
Date: Wednesday, March 16, 2022 Minute 14
"That's sustained…"

We went to the bouncing balloon (Red balloon from last week. The nunchuks were not available)

Although this balloon had become significantly deflated over the course of the week, Kino displayed retained improved bouncing balloon activity.

"That's better," Kino asserted. "That's sustained..."

CHAPTER FIFTY-SEVEN

Subject: Qi Gong in the Treatment of TBI – 5th training session
Date: Wednesday, March 16, 2022 Minute 16
Neurologic exam "…a beautiful thing…"

Before moving to Qi Gong treatment, Bill suggested a more complete neurologic exam be performed. As one who had once aspired to become a Neurologist, I was happy to comply, as I still regarded the neurologic exam like an opportunity to open the hood on the human machine and examine all the gears and wires and circuits.

First, I assessed Kino's reflexes, which were hyperactive (termed, 'hyperreflexia') for the left side.

Kino was surprised by this, commenting that it was his expectation that the reflexes on that side would be impaired.

"Because that's the side of the body that was affected by the TBI," he said. "So, I'd expect the reflexes there to be less."

But that wasn't the way the nervous system worked: The brain works to make reflex responses smoother and more relaxed. Hence, when brain cells die or get damaged, the reflexes become more excitatory, as we saw with him.

Next, an evaluation for subtle weakness was performed. For this, Kino was asked to stretch out both arms with the palms facing up, then keep them in this position with his eyes closed. In Kino's case, his left arm drifted downwards slightly (in what is referred to as 'pronator drift'), again, consistent with his right sided brain injury.

In muscular strength testing, Kino displayed subtle weakness for the muscles of the left side, which was notable for the presence of 'giveaway' weakness (which I'll describe in detail shortly).

Kino commented that he had never had a neurologic exam with muscular testing, despite having been evaluated by not one but two different neurologists since his TBI.

"So, I appreciate it," he said, "because it's kind of something I wanted to know."

Indeed, when I later reviewed the notes from these neurologists, I thought their exams were cursory at best.

Other neurologic testing was discussed (like EMG and nerve conduction study) to evaluate for electrophysiology changes before and after Qi Gong? Bill also raise the possibility of an EEG to evaluate for brainwave activity?

Bill questioned what level of the nervous system we were working on in these Qi Gong treatments?

"Is it following the spinal nerve path?" he asked. " Or is it following the peripheral nerve path? Or is it following something more in the brain where the motor activity is generated?"

Or in the brain where sensation is registered? I wondered.

"Because I'm sitting over here and seeing that the C7 and C8 areas are affected," Bill continued - This based on the sensory exam and Kino's tense numbness at the middle finger). "It would be nice to have something with more objective information to back it up - that would tell us, 'Is this originating back at the brain or somewhere along the spine or the peripheral nerve?' And then we could see where the change happens, and it would be a beautiful thing...

Of note, among the reason I left Neurology was it all seemed so morbid. Like I was so fascinated for these poor people I couldn't help.

"I wish I was the least interesting person in the world," one patient with a neurologic disorder told me.

But in caring for Kino with neurologic deficits, there was this opportunity to determine real objective findings with Qi Gong.

Maybe that's the reason I went so deep into neurology in the first place. And there was a reason that I should come back to medical school after my bio energy experience and be drawn to neurology.

Hence, it crossed my mind that, once again, maybe I got a break that I didn't wind up with that huge new position in addiction, because really I think that the best study is in attempting to find effectiveness in the use of Qi Gong might reside in treating patients with neurologic deficits... Like Kino.

The results with him are better than I've seen with anyone. And that's because they're so definite. At the start of the session, he had neurologic deficits. At the end of the session, those neurologic difficulties were improved and the deficits were less.

Essentially everything else that I'll be asked to do, will have a subjective component. Pain. Addiction.

But in caring for patients with neurologic deficits, then there's the possibility of real objective findings.

Maybe that's the reason I went so deep into neurology in the first place. And there was a reason that I should come back to medical school after my bio energy experience and be drawn to neurology.

CHAPTER FIFTY-EIGHT

Subject: Qi Gong in the Treatment of TBI – 5th training session
Date: Wednesday, March 16, 2022 Minute 32
"...energetically magnetizing every little fiber..."

Initiating Qi Gong treatment, I scanned for an energy disturbances, then invited Bill to attempt to perceive energy over Kino's left side. I especially want him to attempt to find an energy vector that correlated with Kino's left upper back discomfort.

After Bill located it, Kino commented that he was also feeling something.

"I don't know what you're doing, Mr. Miyagi," Kino said, referencing the movie, *The Karate Kid*, "but it's getting warm back there."

Bill attempted to release the energy strain.

"It's interesting," Bill commented. "It feels like it has a spin to it."

He commented that he had not had that kind of perception before.

"But this one seemed like it wanted to spin," he repeated.

I said that was not unusual, and referred to how I often go spinning about the room as I followed energy paths.

I asked Bill if he followed that energetic spinning sensation three dimensional in his mind? He said he had, as opposed to my approach to doing this two dimensionally.

"Well, Mr. Miyagi, it's a very strange phenomenon," Kino offered. "It was first feeling really warm, and then with such finesse, it feels like you're somehow energetically magnetizing every little fiber in my back right there..."

CHAPTER FIFTY-NINE

Subject: Qi Gong in the Treatment of TBI – 5th training session
Date: Wednesday, March 16, 2022 Minute 37
"Much better…"

After Bill finished, I checked the energy at Kino's back; the previous energy imbalance at his upper back was completely neutralized.

As it happened, I perceived an energy strain at Kino's lower back, which was subtle, so I decided to follow it and it, in turn, sent me spinning somewhat in my usual two dimensionally fashion.

I inquired with Kino about his backache discomfort? In response, Kino described having an energy experience with Bill and then me.

"I noticed the warmth and gravitational pull," Kino said of Bill. "And then whatever you did became more about a pull that shifted away from pinching on the left side of my back, till it was less and got centered and even and warm.

"And then Dr. Yanuck took over, and I took a deep breath, and the sensation of the little pinches was less, so that I was kind of healed muscularly."

He stretched.

"Much better," Kino said. "Much better..."

CHAPTER SIXTY

Subject: Qi Gong in the Treatment of TBI – 5th training session
Date: Wednesday, March 16, 2022 Minute 43
"...far and wide..."

I perceived energy movement along the left side of Kino's body from his head down his arm and out, and asked Bill to check and see what he found?

Bill perceived the energy movement and then followed it a significant distance from Kino's body.

"How far will it go out?" he asked.

I explained that in following the energy's path during the bioenergy treatment phase, it is not impossible that it will lead you far and wide. I shared that early in my training, there was one occasion when one recipient's energy path extended beyond the confines of the room I was performing bioenergy in! This happened while I was working with Lena (mother of my friend Liz). When Lena came to visit us in Washington, D.C., I noticed she walked with an abnormal, wobbling, side-to-side gait. When asked how long she'd had the problem, she responded, "I couldn't say. For years. Maybe it was from having six children?" Scanning Lena, I found that the energy emanating from her filled the room in a way I'd never experienced before. Following the path of the energy took me from wall to wall, requiring chairs to reach high enough, and opening windows to pursue its path outside. In the meantime, Lena (who suffered from narcolepsy) had fallen asleep.

"Should I wake her?" Liz asked.

I suggested we let her sleep, especially as the pursuit of these energy disturbances (which was taking me onto chairs and through windows) was leaving me not a little embarrassed.

Lena awoke shortly after I'd finished. When she got up from the couch, she walked across the room with no trace of her earlier wobble.

"Mom, you're walking straight!" Liz called out.

For the rest of her visit Lena walked without difficulty. At the airport on her way to her flight back home, she walked the length of the concourse as straight as an arrow. Even when we visited her in Rhode Island months later, she was still walking without any trace of wobble.

When I confided this experience to Dr. Rind, he responded with the following advice: "You don't have to physically follow the energy everywhere it goes. You could follow it in three dimensions in your mind without moving... After locating the strain pattern, follow its pull. Does it suck you in? Does it push you away? Stand still, and experience where it's going. This way, you can arrive at a three-dimensional understanding of the pulls produced by the trauma."

Nevertheless (perhaps because of the inspiring results achieved for Lena), it would be years before I embraced my mentor's recommendation, and, really, I still prefer the practice of physically following the path of energy strain...

CHAPTER SIXTY-ONE

Subject: Qi Gong in the Treatment of TBI – 5th training session
Date: Wednesday, March 16, 2022 Minute 47

I posed the question, Why would we be finding so much in the way of energy disturbances on Kino's left side when it would seem that the primary source of Kino's difficulties related to strength and coordination and sensation had to do with what happened to the right side of his brain?

I wondered if this might be because, while Kino was in a coma, there might have been a disconnect between the peripheral nerves and the brain? Afterall, while he was in a coma, the brain was not feeding messages to those parts of his body. Indeed, even after the coma, given the injury, the brain might not have been feeding significant signals to that part of the body. And in that way, the peripheral nerves might have shut down because they were not receiving that input?

And perhaps now this Qi Gong work was bridging that disconnect? Opening the peripheral nerves to signals from the brain, which it had perhaps not received and thereby shutdown?

As though the energy treatments were relating a message to those peripheral nerves, so to say, 'I know that the system was down for a while, but now the system is up, so that it's time to become functional again.'

And that's why it might be that we were working with the left side so much… Because we were working with peripheral nerves that had shut themselves off because they'd expected there to have been irreparable damage at the level of the brain...

CHAPTER SIXTY-TWO

Subject: Qi Gong in the Treatment of TBI – 5th training session
Date: Wednesday, March 16, 2022 Minute 48
"More responsive…"

I noted that (unlike the last session) Kino had not described any tingling or twitching in his hands during this session.

When I inquired about this, Kino reflected for a long time and examined his hands; he indicated that those sensations had not been his experience this time, and rubbing his fingers, he noted that it was the feeling of "shocking" (on stimulation of the fingers) that was his predominant experience this time.

I inquired if the Qi Gong treatments were making a difference in his daily life? Kino indicated that he noticed the improvements in sensation with his left hand while driving.

"I like to drive with just one hand," he said. "With my [left] hand around the steering wheel, I could feel the little notches. I could feel a little bit more, but it's not so easy as with the right, but I can still grab it. I can still drive straight with the left hand. So, it's better. It's more responsive."

He commented about something that he said from last week about riding a bike, he described better balance on his bicycle, so that he could turn and look back at his girlfriend and still ride his bike in a forward direction.

"I'm still steady, centered," he said. "So, I think that's a positive, good thing from this…"

CHAPTER SIXTY-THREE

Subject: Qi Gong in the Treatment of TBI – 5th training session
Date: Wednesday, March 16, 2022 Minute 59
Heart chakra

Performing a scan over Kino, I noted an energy disturbance at the center of his chest, in a location that I would describe is the 'heart chakra.'

Upon bringing it to Bill's attention, he evaluated for it, as well; starting from the top of Kino's head, Bill scanned over Kino's midline. Afterwards, he indicated he perceived energy from several chakra points, starting at the top of Kino's head.

I went back and located the active chakras: Starting with the third eye chakra, I followed its energy path with my right hand. Next, I went to the throat chakra with my left hand, and followed its path. That chakra released with relative ease, so I re-use the left hand to follow the heart chakra energy. Of note, it was only with the heart chakra that I felt energy from a distance (in the ether level), whereas the others I perceived the energy closer to the body.

Afterwards, I invited Bill to check the energy is there again.

"Much more smooth," he said. "This one [He said indicated the third eye chakra] I don't even feel."

Of the heart chakra, he also indicated a change, saying, "It's moving. It's flowing."

I shared how it was that as I was working on Kino's heart chakra, I experienced a feeling of euphoria.

"Yeah, I could see that," Bill said. "A release… A relief type of feeling."

Of note, in reviewing the recording of this session, I visibly observed my chest go from it usual shallow and sunken state to being open and expanded. Observing the difference in our physiques (How open-chested Kino was, compared to my sunken chest), I considered his ease and comfort with himself, compared with my usually pressured, nervous, rushed state of being, and thought I could benefit from Kino's energy that way, and probably had over the course of the energy interaction just now, while working with his heart chakra…

CHAPTER SIXTY-FOUR

Subject: Qi Gong in the Treatment of TBI – 5th training session
Date: Wednesday, March 16, 2022 Minute 1:03
Parting thoughts…

Bill indicated that he had to leave. Before departing he described the session as "very productive", in particular, citing the "energy spin" experience he'd had at the beginning of the Qi Gong treatment.

"That was neat," he said.

Kino chimed in, saying that he had heard of chakras, but did not have an understanding of them? I briefly described chakras as energy centers and would have elaborated, but Kino essentially deferred, saying, "It's OK, doc. I'm happy to be the subject here..."

At essentially that moment, I felt the energy evaporate from my hands, so to suggest that the Qi Gong treatment was done.

With that, we moved to re-evaluate, starting with reviewing his motor skills with the bouncing balloon.

The use of this bouncing balloon was rather difficult with the left hand. In particular, in order to control the bouncing, Kino was straining at muscles of the upper chest and shoulder.

"I have to tense my muscles and keep them in a tense mode," he indicated of the left hand. "Whereas [with the right hand), no tenseness."

Still, he felt there was improvement.

"It's much improved," he asserted, and added that he thought it was a "right hand dominant thing."

In addition, Kino indicated that he had done something today that he hadn't in four years.

"A push-up with a clap in the middle," he said. "I did it last in front of Emily on our wedding day. That's the very last time until today that I accomplished one clap after I did ten pushups. I think that has to do with this. Because I couldn't bring my hands up quick enough to clap. And now I can. So, thank you..."

CHAPTER SIXTY-FIVE

Subject: Qi Gong in the Treatment of TBI – 5th training session
Date: Wednesday, March 16, 2022 Minute 1:08

Next, we went to the sensory exam. He indicated that this time the sensation of light touch was more similar between the two hands, with less of the electrical feeling.

"It felt very much the same," he said. "It's an improvement."

Still, the left middle finger continued to have less sensation, as well as a persistent electrical feeling in response to light touch.

This same pattern of improvement for all left-hand digits except middle continued for sensory exams involving pinprick and vibration...

CHAPTER SIXTY-SIX

Subject: Qi Gong in the Treatment of TBI – 5th training session
Date: Wednesday, March 16, 2022 Minute 1:13

I re-evaluated his muscular strength: Although there was some persistent biceps weakness on the left side, his triceps strength was significantly improved. This pattern of improved strength continued for wrist extension for the left, then wrist flexion, then finger extension, then finger flexion.

Later, Kino would note that when he bench-pressed at home, he had difficulty for the left side, saying, "I do have a lot more trouble getting it up on my left."

Re-evaluating pronator drift, this was also improved, with less lowering of his left hand.

Something that I hadn't recorded previously was rapid alternating movements, which I had previously noted was a difficulty for Kino (and a significant oversight on my part for having not evaluated it at the beginning of the session), because it was remarkably improved now. Previously, his right arm would spin around in around his left (like a planet's orbit about the sun). This time the two were spinning around each other with relatively equal speed. Meanwhile, I thought left-sided weakness might be a factor in the rapid alternating movement disparity, because the longer that Kino performed the exercise, the more the equality between the two sides diminished and the more the left-side deficits showed up. This fatigue factor was probably also at the heart of the bouncing balloon difficulty observed earlier.

For expanded finger-to-nose testing, Kino displayed some slowness and hesitation for the left side.

"As I was going out," Kino noted, "I had a bit of a question mark. It wasn't just a straight shot. A little bit of question mark..."

CHAPTER SIXTY-SEVEN

Subject: Qi Gong in the Treatment of TBI – 5th training session
Date: Wednesday, March 16, 2022 Minute 1:20

Kino inquired about the other Veteran with traumatic brain injury who'd received a Qi Gong session, saying that he would be interested in comparing the benefit she received with those that he received from Qi Gong?

"Because I am receiving a different therapy than I imagine anyone else in the world has," he said. "And just the differences and similarities of our injuries and what difference do we receive from the same treatment would be interesting to know."

Yes, Kino was rather unique in his TBI, as most persons don't suffer from focal neurologic deficits from TBI as he had.

Meanwhile, I was, indeed, inspired to work with more patients with traumatic brain injury having observed the results and improvements that Kino was achieving with Qi Gong...

CHAPTER SIXTY-EIGHT

Subject: Qi Gong in the Treatment of TBI – 5th training session
Date: Wednesday, March 16, 2022 Minute 1:20

Finally, I offered to share how I performed Qi Gong self-practice; in particular, the muscular releases that I experienced in the course of that self-practice. It happened with the continued bioenergy/Qi Gong practice (especially in the time that I'd worked with my father a couple of years ago), I had reached a higher level in my own self-healing, such that the crippling spasms/trigger points in my body would nearly automatically start to release when I entered a 'Qi Gong-state.'

Basically, it worked like this: Putting myself in a neutral position, I almost immediately experienced trigger point releases. This was most easily accomplished in the supine position, but could also happen while sitting and standing. The releases are essentially involuntary, and the resulting contractions could appear almost violent: when it involves the muscles around my midback, their contractions around my ribcage produce forced exhalation; other times I'll go flopping around like a proverbial fish! As to why these releases are so 'explosive', the feeling is it's because these muscles are locked in spasm, so to be effectively 'set in cement.'

"And once they're 'cemented'," a colleague said, "the only way you can break out of it, is to break the cement."

I believe the 'cement' is the muscle myofibrils – the actin and myosin – which are locked into one into one big spasm. That's what a trigger point is! And you need significant energy to elicit the 'jump signs' to unlock them, so that afterwards those filaments will slide by each other and let the muscle relax. That's how you break the cement! The explosions are basically large jump signs in which the actin and myosin disengage by contracting to unhinge before spontaneously releasing.

Nevertheless, despite the explosiveness of these spontaneous contractions ('jump signs'), the process was entirely painless, which I believe is because pain is related to inflammation, and where these injuries are so old (and the 'cement' laid down so long ago), there's no inflammation to be had. It's just releases that are happening. So, as startling as the jump signs appear, there's no pain whatsoever.

In summary, this process works to release trigger points that can't otherwise be released, so to free up those muscles for use. And as more of these muscles move from a dysfunctional state to one of function, I become a better vessel of healing. Because I'm more open, my system is working better and I can serve as a better channel for the healing energy of the universe to move through me, so to help another. The spontaneous release process can go on for seconds, minutes or hours, though I can consciously stop it at any moment. After undergoing these releases, it never fails that I feel light, relaxed, grounded and significantly more agile.

But despite my enthusiasm for sharing this phenomenon with the others, it was felt best that we wait till Bill was with us again, so it was mutually decided to save it for next time (which led me to problems, because I wound up rushing the process of re-evaluating Kino. I'll detail that in the discussion of the next Qi Gong session)...

CHAPTER SIXTY-NINE

"Flow"

During the night after the Qi Gong session, I was hearing Bill's voice in my head.

"It's a different flow..." "It's moving. It's flowing..."

Then, I sat up bolt upright in bed: I suddenly understood something – It had to do with what Bill was saying and conveying about "flow", and engendered a great understanding of the importance of the work we were doing than I had ever before imagined! Indeed, it spoke to a radical new understanding and appreciation for the energetics circulation.

Just as the blood flows through the veins and arteries and capillaries of the the body to nourish the tissues, so does the energetic circulation work that way. We (Bill and I and any other good energy healer) might as well be as Cardiologists and Vascular surgeons of the energetic circulation, unblocking that circulation and facilitating virtual energetic stents, so to re-establish the flow of energy in the body.

Bioenergy/Qi Gong is more than just about releasing energy strains and disturbances, I realized. It's facilitating and promoting the energetic circulation!

And, the odd thing was, I'd always known this: Any book I'd ever written about bioenergy/Qi Gong had always begun with the same two sentences:

"In its normal state the human energy field flows in a regular, even pattern. When the body sustains trauma, though, blockages in the energetic circulation develop that can manifest in physical disease."

But I wasn't until this moment that I'd put it all together.

Where the energetic circulation is blocked and not moving, the energy is stuck. It's like the claudication (i.e., the narrowing) of a blood vessel: The energy can't move; The energy can't adequately perfuse the tissues. Energy disturbances might as well be the equivalent of coronary artery disease. You don't have the energy flow you need, so the body is weak, deteriorating and potentially dying! Then, you need energy healing, so to facilitate and correct that blockage in the energetic circulation! You need this for health!

It's what was probably going on in my muscles. That's why my acupuncturist says of them that when he goes through them with a needle, it's as though they're hollow, and there isn't any Chi being released. It's because there's an inadequacy of Chi flow there. It's not a problem of the muscles, it's a problem of energy flow and the energetic circulation. It's because the Qi is not getting there!

That's why when I perform my Qi Gong self-practice, I experience muscular releases all over in my core body (back and trunk), but I don't experience those releases over my distant sties (like my legs and feet). It's because there's not enough energy flow to feed the tissues of those more distant body parts, so to permit and facilitate those muscular releases.

Hence, as well as blood flow, you need energy flow!...

Then, I dreamt that I was evaluating a patient with a recent stroke. The case was complicated because the patient was comatose, and performing the neurologic exam, I found his main deficits were on his right side.

Then, the patient became awake and alert and talked about having had a previous stroke affecting his left side. I listened to him, but didn't perform a follow-up examination.

Documenting my findings, a second year Neurology Resident came by and said that he'd been sent to perform a full evaluation on the patient.

"But maybe I don't need to," he added, "because you've already done one."

I shared my findings, then described my conversation with the patient.

"Did you check whether he could voluntarily grasp item with his left hand?" the Resident asked.

Admitting that I hadn't, I chastised myself for having not done so...

Awakening from the dream, I considered the Qi Gong project and the fact that until today I had not performed a thorough neurologic exam on Kino.

Why hadn't I done it before? I thought. Why hadn't I been more thorough? Was it because I was so swept up with Kino's improvements that it had just become a matter of saying, "Kino, what do you want to work on today?" and just going with the flow of what Kino wanted and we'd already started, so that all I wanted to do was focus on the bouncing ball and nunchuks, and I didn't even want to introduce anything else?

Or was there more to it than that? Like maybe the fact that it was ingrained in me to expect that patients with neurologic deficits didn't get better?

"That's why I left Neurology in the first place," I thought.

Let me elaborate: I had plans to become a Neurologist. Even after I'd spearheaded the development of a cancer vaccine (and authored an entire doctorate on its development) putting me in well onto the road of becoming an oncologist, I fell in love with a neurologic exam. It felt like opening the hood of the human machine and getting to see how all the gears and circuits worked. So enamored was I of this skill that I changed course to become a neurologist!

But my Neurology Residency was harsh and woke me up to the harsh nature of the profession, in general: Here I was finding these patients so fascinating, and, for them, they wished they were the least interesting people on earth! Over time, I was left feeling that mine was a morbid fascination, at my patient's expense. Because, in general, there was nothing that could be done for them. The damage has been done. They weren't going to recover.

And, in retrospect, I believe I took that Neurology training into the Qi Gong project, such that the reason I didn't evaluate Kino neurologically to assess for neurologic deficits to improve was because I didn't believe it was possible.

"That's impossible," the voice in my head was probably telling me. "Patients don't recover from neurologic injury like this. For the most part, they only get worse."

A personal bias conditioned in me based on years of training in conventional Neurology - Just as the vast majority of my colleagues were conditioned not to believe in energy healing modalities like bioenergy and Qi Gong).

So, as well as swimming against the stream of conventional medicine biases, I was also fighting the current where my prior

training was concerned, planted in me over years of training that I had received in this area.

Then, I was reminded of a dream that I had in medical school, while I was caring for my anatomy professor who was dying of cancer: I dreamt that I was going into this dark cave and descending and descending and descending deeper into it and all there was, was gloom.

And then I heard someone calling to me to come out of that cave and leave all that gloom.

And (long story short) I stepped into the light...

And so I left the Neurology Residency, and went into Internal Medicine, where I could mostly assist patients with every kind of condition, facilitating their health and offering some hope.

And now I wondered that my friend, my coworker, my teammate, wasn't offering me the chance to find my way back to Neurology – to the study of conditions that I found most fascinating – but without all the gloom, because by applying my passion, my calling in life to – Energy Medicine – I could help patients with neurologic conditions and deficits?...

CHAPTER SEVENTY

Subject: Qi Gong in the Treatment of TBI - 6th training session
Date: Wednesday, March 23, 2022 Minute 0:00
Broken clavicle

We began the Qi Gong session with Kino performing the bouncing balloon exercise. Kino made the point that it required a "flick of the wrist," for which he had no problem with the right hand, but significant difficulty with the left.

"It's all coming from here," he said, indicating his left shoulder.

Indeed, his movement at the left shoulder appeared tense, constrained and restricted. Furthermore, Kino described feelings of fatigue while performing the activity with his left, whereas there was no such fatigue for his right side.

Kino raised the point that he'd sustained a broken left clavicle not long after the TBI and wondered if that could have something to do with the left shoulder difficulty?

Pulling down on his shirt, he displayed an obvious deformity and misalignment in the bone, mid-clavicle.

"I'm wondering if that has any part in this?" he asked.

He shared how it was that he had elected not to undergo surgical repair of the broken clavicle.

"So, it's not quite lined up to allow free movement at the shoulder," he said and wondered if bioenergy/Qi Gong could help?

I agreed and felt that treatment of likely energy disturbances at the clavicle would be the focus of the session.

Little did I know that the session would hold so much more…

CHAPTER SEVENTY-ONE

Subject: Qi Gong in the Treatment of TBI - 6th training session
Date: Thursday, March 17, 2022 Minute 10
"...flick of the wrist."

Going to the nunchuks, Kino again indicated that with this exercise, too, was a matter of a "flick of the wrist."

He spun them with both hands and, again, there was the tenseness in his left shoulder.

"But this is so much better than what I could do," he acknowledged.

Neurological exam was performed next:

Pronator drift was improved, with no notable lowering of his left hand.

"I feel really steady," Kino commented.

Coordination was improved for finger to nose for his left side, such that he displayed less hesitation.

Rapid alternating movements were also improved and relatively equal between the two sides.

Evaluation of reflexes showed persistent hyperreflexia on the left side for both upper and lower extremities.

"I felt a lot more 'reflex' on that left versus right," Kino acknowledged. "It's weird to me, because I feel like that's where I have the problem?"

I explained that it actually did make sense, and that contralateral hyperreflexia was a mark of brain injury. Hence, where he had the traumatic brain injury on the right side, it would be expected that the reflexes on the left would be affected.

Of note, the site of greatest hyperreflexia was at the brachioradialis muscle (in the forearm, near the left wrist), such that more than just responding with movement at the arm, his whole hand flexed…

CHAPTER SEVENTY-TWO

Subject: Qi Gong in the Treatment of TBI - 6th training session
Date: Wednesday, March 23, 2022 Minute 21

Kino had commented he felt his sensation had continued to be improved for the fingers of his affected left hand.

"The finger numbness is better," he said. "Not quite fixed."

On sensory testing, Kino indicated that his perception of light touch was relatively equal between the two hands, and without the electrical feeling they had previously been there.

Indeed, today, the electrical feeling was limited to the middle finger.

This pattern continued for pinprick, vibration and temperature testing, as well…

CHAPTER SEVENTY-THREE

Subject: Qi Gong in the Treatment of TBI - 6th training session
Date: Wednesday, March 23, 2022 Minute 28

Muscular testing showed some persistent giveaway weakness for the muscles of the left side of his body.

"It was like it took a second," Kino described. "Like, 'Here it comes.'"

Yes, as though it took his brain needed to process the force I was applying before it triggered the muscular response needed to resist.

'Giveaway weakness' is generally considered a 'functional' form of weakness; that is, not true weakness, though not anything the person is actively doing or consciously aware. This form of weakness can stem from a nerve conduction block (as occasionally seen in Multiple Sclerosis patients when they describe their legs not moving as fast as their brains are signaling). Moreover, I thought Kino weakness this way was related to the residual 'Hemineglect' that he experienced with the TBI.

Hemineglect is a disabling condition that commonly follows brain damage, in which patients fail to be aware of items and parts of their own body on the affected side.

In Kino's case, I'd witness his hemineglect up close and personal back when he was in the hospital recovering from the TBI: During those nights that I'd sit with him, I observed that (as incapacitated as he was), Kino still had the presence of mind to want to communicate with friends and family. Like a lot of his, his chief tool for doing this was his cellphone; and as his left hand was completely useless at that time, he'd type his texts entirely with the right (mostly his right thumb), completely neglecting the use of the left.

Whole books had been written on the subject of hemineglect; in particular, Oliver Sacks' classic, 'A Leg to Stand On', in which the author described his own difficulties overcoming the condition.

Indeed, in a later Qi Gong session, I would describe this book in detail, as I introduced issues that Dr. Sacks' contended with that were not dissimilar from those Kino was facing. That was later on, when another mental health staff member (Nancy) joined us and would make significant contributions in Kino's Qi Gong treatment and described in the planned subsequent work titled, *Shot of Love...*

CHAPTER SEVENTY-FOUR

Subject: Qi Gong in the Treatment of TBI - 6th training session
Date: Wednesday, March 23, 2022 Minute 33.

Moving to the Qi Gong therapy aspect of the session, I scanned Kino's left side energetically and perceived multiple energy vectors at his head and shoulder.

Given this finding, I introduced the concept of the Key Lesion, which goes like this: Although, in general, the primary source of most energy imbalances is the place where it is initially perceived. However, if you find that an energy disturbance is not responding to your attempts to neutralized it, then consider holding a hand there, and, with the other, scan the rest of the body. If you then find that an energy disturbance at a distant site that neutralizes the energy at the first, then you've probably encountered the primary lesion there. Hence, every so often you will encounter an energy vector that does not respond to your attempts at neutralizing it. This is likely because this is not the key lesion (or primary lesion) that holds the key to healing and really requires your attention. When this happens, look for a second energy disturbance and determine if there is a relationship between them. This is done by keeping your hand over the first energy vector and then scanning for and locating a second energy vector with your other hand. If there is a relationship between the two energy vectors, then the energy from the first one will drop off, such that you'll be left only feeling energy from the second – because the retained energy of the trauma is really held at that second energy vector, and the first was just a downstream effect and not the true source.

This was a rather advanced topic and really I didn't know if it was all that apropos.

Nevertheless, Bill (being the great student of this practice that he was) was game to give it a try; when he did, he found that the energy over Kino's shoulder faded when his other hand perceived energy over Kino's head.

"Initially I felt it at both spots," He said. "The parietal region [of the head] and his shoulder. Then, the parietal region was hot, and the shoulder was not."

This would suggest that the energy disturbance over the head was the key lesion.

Returning to Kino and evaluating this myself, I noted a similar phenomenon and invited Bill to treat the lesion.

In turn, Bill worked for a long time to release the energy disturbance at Kino's head, but ultimately stopped, indicating that he was having difficulty and saying "it was not cooling down like it had before."

I attempted a release the energy disturbance: Within a minute, I felt it squarely in my hand, and invited Bill to go back and check for any difference.

"The shoulder has cooled off," Bill acknowledged…

CHAPTER SEVENTY-FIVE

Subject: Qi Gong in the Treatment of TBI - 6th training session
Date: Wednesday, March 23, 2022 Minute 45
Crown Chakra

Bill perceived energy at the top of Kino's head. Evaluating the area myself, I confirmed this and wondered aloud if this might be related to Kino's 'crown chakra' and launched into a rather long discourse on the subject.

The crown chakra (or seventh chakra) occurs at the vertex of the head. This chakra theoretically connects us with the universe and kindles our desire for spirituality ideals like unconditional love.

In my experience, imbalances at the crown chakra occur when traumatic experiences cause us to wall ourselves off from others, and relatively common for it to be activated after reconciling a significant energy disturbance, especially those involving other chakra imbalances.

Typically, when my crown chakra opens, I feel a certain sense of euphoria (accompanied by a feeling of awe and reverence) and feel connected with the universe and everything around me.

I shared the story of my crown chakra experience that occurred after caring for first love's mother, saying that when my work was done and it was time to leave Bubbles and her family, I was expecting it to be as difficult (as it had always, being that I loved them so much). Hence, stepping onto that departing Greyhound bus and taking a seat in the back, I drew a deep breath and wondered, 'When is it going to hit? The remorse and sadness?'

Then, as the bus drove off, I became aware of an emerging feeling: It wasn't the familiar emptiness and hollowness in my chest, but, rather, a sensation of energy, starting at my head till beaming and overflowing to every part of me, so that I was enveloped in a cocoon of energy, fuller and more expansive than anything I'd ever experienced before!

My thought at the time was, 'I've honored something. I've shown some great respect. It's something simple, yet wonderful. It reaches to the core of my being – God is love...'

And since then, I've referred to this as my 'God is Love' experience.

I continued by sharing about an experience guided self-practice with a person who

I'll refer to here as K. K described a childhood filled with horrific physical and mental abuse, from which he was still suffering. It happened that K only lived about a hundred miles away from me, so I suggested we meet in-person. However, he was insistent that we attempt a guided self-practice session, saying that he just had a feeling that 'remote healing' would be helpful to him. Feeling it couldn't do any harm, I agreed and focused on him and his life story and opened myself to any energy I might be sensing. In time, energy filled my hands as I followed it in the directions that it took them. Then, some minutes later, I experienced a feeling of energy at my head, as though tethering me between the crown chakra and the universe, and kindling the memory of the 'God is Love' experience from twenty-five years before.

In sum, I told Bill and Kino that this was essentially a long way of saying that when it came to the chakras, you might have a different energy experience than what you expect and wind up opening up the chakras, so to release significant retained energy of trauma, and it could become more intense at first before all of that energy is finally released; thereby, possibly explaining how it was that Bill experienced of the energy a Kino's head "heating up" at first, rather that the usual pattern of just moving off and fading, as it flowed way.

"Which isn't a bad thing," I asserted. "Because sometimes the chakras do need to open up and release a lot of retain energy, so to realign and facilitate healing…"

CHAPTER SEVENTY-SIX

Subject: Qi Gong in the Treatment of TBI - 6th training session
Date: Wednesday, March 23, 2022 Minute 50

By this time the energy had led me back to Kino, such that I was right where I'd begun, at his left shoulder and emitting healing energy back to him.

"I'm getting really relaxed," he commented. "And it's like, I don't really know what the heck you guys are talking about, but I get it a little. It's like guys are riding a wave of common language, and I'm the water."

"And as you're moving around me," he continued, "I felt warmth in different areas, and I wonder if you can see that I'm swaying forward and backwards and left and right, and it's just happening."

Even on reviewing the recording, I did not perceive him moving. It must be very minute.

"And I'm having a tough time staying still with whatever you're doing with your energy, my energy, whatever," he said.

Kino indicated that he was experiencing goosebumps.

"It's not entirely cold in here," he said.

I asked if he was uncomfortable, but he said, "I'm fine."

I wondered if an energy experience (specifically, the release of retained energy of trauma) was the source of the goosebumps?...

CHAPTER SEVENTY-SEVEN

Subject: Qi Gong in the Treatment of TBI - 6th training session
Date: Wednesday, March 23, 2022 Minute 57

Noting an intense energy radiating from Kino‘s fingers, I invited Bill to evaluate over the area without specifically telling him what to look for.

“It’s interesting,” Bill commented. “Previous times I remember it being more at his palms. This time it was at his fingers.”

Attempting energy release there, I shared my thoughts that the electrical sensation Kino was experiencing at the fingers upon sensory stimulation might be related to some ‘reawakening’ of the nerves, and the nervous system working on the “re-wiring” and “connecting the circuits”; getting everything integrated, such that we were working to facilitate that by treating the energetics circulation and corrected any imbalances there and facilitating the normal flow of energy within the body mind.

I commented that the energy disturbances were not the same as they’ve been in the beginning: In the beginning they’d been more obvious, and now they were more subtle (and being that Kino energy disturbances were more or less subtle from the start, then these were really subtle!).

Still, I wasn’t perceiving an energy shell around Kino, plus I was going to continue to work on those energy disturbances, despite how subtle they work…

CHAPTER SEVENTY-EIGHT

Subject: Qi Gong in the Treatment of TBI - 6th training session
Date: Wednesday, March 23, 2022 Minute 1:09

The energy having left me, signaling the completion of the treatment session.

In turn, I asked if we should reevaluate and look for any changes in his exam?

Kino ran his fingers over each other for both hands.

"I rub my fingers," he said, "and I feel there's a difference.

"In this hand [right, unaffected], I feel the vibration of fingerprints sliding across each other. In his hand [affected left], there's vibration and it's a little electrical, but nonetheless, I can feel more.

"So, yeah, I want to see you, because I can see you guys are doing the magic of Qi Gong and bioenergy, and I just feel affected."

Perform the sensory exam, I began with evaluation for light touch.

Kino felt there was improvement.

"I think there is a difference," he said. "They felt more similar."

Pinprick was similar, with Kino commenting, "It feels different. It feels more the same than different."

Kino showed improvement for the vibration sensation, especially for his densely affected left middle finger.

"A dull vibrating," he said of the finger. "No shocking. Yeah, there's a difference."

Going to the bouncing balloon, Kino showed significant improvement.

"A lot more wrist," he said. "Less of a fatigue. Some improvement."

He indicated that he was still using some shoulder on the left side.

"But overall improved," he asserted.

Next was the nunchuks. Here he performed the exercise with his left shoulder more open (and less constrained) and he indicated significantly less fatigue…

CHAPTER SEVENTY-NINE

Subject: Qi Gong in the Treatment of TBI - 6th training session
Date: Wednesday, March 23, 2022 Minute 1:20
"Syncing"

I offered to demonstrate the muscular releases that occur when I perform Qi Gong self-practice.

Earlier, I'd shared how it was that performing these Qi Gong sessions was having beneficial effects on me, such that when I leave these sessions, my Qi Gong self-practice is more intense, with significant muscular releases.

I shared my feelings that one of the beauties of this work was that as well as helping someone else, in general of this work was helpful to the Qi Gong practitioner, as well.

"Usually we're not good at scanning ourselves," I said. "I mean - How are we going to find energy disturbances when we are reverberating at the same energy?

"But in performing this work, it gets you in tune with your energetic system."

Indeed, I believed that the energy of the patient reaches back into the practitioner, so to facilitate healing in those places where energy disturbances exist in the practitioner.

I said that at times my body would go flopping around like a fish out of water, and explained that if that were to happen, not be worried that I was experiencing anything like seizures, as I was completely awake and cognizant of my surroundings; and these were the manifestations of "jump signs", whereby a short contraction was needed to release the spastic overlap of interconnecting actin and myosin fibrils, before eliciting a significant release, with the fibrils just slid over each other.

I continue that this was a pleasurable experience, and usually I felt more relaxed afterwards.

Laying supine on the examination table, I demonstrated for the group these muscular releases to the extent that my body was able to within the small confines of the table.

Afterwards, I, again, stressed how it was that after performing this work, the practitioner might feel some benefits, as well.

"Because the patient is looking to make you an even better vessel of healing," I said. "Just as the practitioner is working on them, they're looking for the kinks in you - where your system isn't quite right – so that they'll tap on your system's shoulder and say, 'Hey, I can help you there,' and then help you."

Indeed, it was my belief that in the process of working with Kino, there was more going on than just tapping into his energetic circulation to "jumpstart" his nervous system: In bioenergy/Qi Gong, I believe the practitioner and patient are not unlike a couple of computers syncing with each other through a fiber optic cable.

Kino's "computer"/nervous system had a problem, such that transmitting neural signals was defective, analogous to having a "corrupted program" that had been damaged by the TBI, so that it wasn't "running" effectively. On the other hand, Bill and my nervous system/"computers" had working neural programs that had not been damaged, so that when we "synced" with Kino (via connecting through the energetic circulation), Kino's nervous system/computer was identifying where it had problems, syncing with our working systems, and correcting those "corrupted/damaged programs" - the information travelling between us via the energetic circulation (just like a couple computers connected by a fiber optic cable) until the self-repair/re-programming was optimally restored and in working order (to the extent that his nervous system had working programs to be corrected) and ready to run again.

And I contended there was even more to this interplay between Kino and Bill and me: I believed that, where he could, Kino's system was giving back to me; that just as a fiber optic cable permits the sharing of information between the connected computers, so does information about energy disturbances travel back-and-forth between healer and healee via the energetic circulation, shuttling information for the purpose of healing and facilitating a dynamic interpersonal link designed to help one another.

"It's just win-win," I declared…

CHAPTER EIGHTY

Subject: Qi Gong in the Treatment of TBI - 6th training session
Date: Wednesday, March 23, 2022 Minute 1:28.
"Energy cleanse"

I shared how it was that my early difficulties with this energetic interplay between patient and practitioner was what got me into Qi Gong in the first place. Early in my training, I'd be performing bioenergy on someone and find that I was experiencing an agonizing 'buzz' (akin to an aching headache) and find that (along with the discomfort) I wasn't able to energetically help the other person. As a result, I contemplated leaving bioenergy altogether; but my friend Liz suggested it might be a matter of me needing to make a personal journey into my own healing and suggested doing this through the practice of Qi Gong.

The typical pattern in Qi Gong training is to first learn the self-maintenance of Qi Gong (or Qi Gong self-practice). Here, rather than an energy healer working on you to attend energy imbalances (as with bioenergy and Medical Qi Gong), one connects with the Universal Chi, so to forge a direct connection with the 'Universal Blueprint' that theoretically contains the knowledge for healing all things (to the extent possible). By energetically tapping into this Universal Blueprint through the practice of Qi Gong, one effectively reboots and jump-starts the system, so to facilitate self-healing.

Ultimately, it was the merging of my bioenergy practice with Qi Gong self-practice that got me beyond my occasional patient difficulties – and much more!

It happened this way: After training in Qi Gong self-practice, I went back to treating patients with bioenergy; Not long after, during a bioenergy session, I encountered a patient who triggered that agonizing buzz feeling. And this time, rather than get discouraged and give up with the patient, I interrupted the bioenergy session to perform a Qi Gong self-practice and energetically attend whatever it was that was coming up in me. Afterwards, I found I felt refreshed and invigorated and then went back to the patient and found that I was now able to help him via bioenergy.

This opened me to a whole new realm of serving as an energy practitioner: I'd learned firsthand that the patients I used to dread were those who had the most to give me – Because they were energetically activating my old wounds!

These patients suffered from a similar energy disturbance as I did: The difference was, mine was chronic and dormant, whereas theirs was active and acute. That ill-at-ease feeling I was experiencing was that old wound being 'activated'; before it had been lying chronic and dormant in my system; the bioenergy session had brought it to the surface, converting it from an inactive, chronic state to one that was active and acute. In general, it is only in this 'activated' state that an energy strain is amenable to healing.

Now, when I encounter a patient who activates my chronic, dormant traumas, I don't even need to interrupt the energy session to perform a Qi Gong self-practice, because it happens automatically; my system simply recognizes that the patient and I possess a similar energy disturbance and then goes about repairing it and healing me.

Listening, Bill nodded.

"It was bringing me back to working with the herbs," he said. "Sometimes when you're doing a cleanse, you get headaches and you don't feel great; but the theory behind that is it's stirring up toxins and you need to flush them out; and you drink a lot of water, and the headache goes away, and you feel better than you did in the first place. Because the toxins have been buried and stuck in your tissues and muscles and fat or whatever, and the cleanse has stirred it up, and in this way it's almost like an energy thing…"

CHAPTER EIGHTY-ONE

Subject: Qi Gong in the Treatment of TBI - 6th training session
Date: Wednesday, March 23, 2022
Summary…

In this session I'd introduced a number of advance topics in energy healing, which could be summarized as follows:

1. The Key Lesion:
2. The seventh chakra or 'crown chakra':
3. Muscle releases in the Qi Gong practitioner:
4. Reawakening old wounds in the Qi Gong practitioner:
5. Reciprocated healing:

In all, Kino was exhibiting levels of neurologic recovery that I couldn't have imagined, making this the most exciting and medically gratifying time of my life…

CHAPTER EIGHTY-TWO

Subject: Qi Gong in the Treatment of TBI – 7th training session
Date: Wednesday, March 30, 2022 Minute 0
"Double Dribble"

In the 7th Qi Gong training session, Kino brought basketball as a new activity to challenge himself.

"It really isn't my thing," he said. "But it's something to objectively measure what's going on here."

He displayed considerable difficulty dribbling with the left hand.

"I'm righthand dominant," he said. "But really in a lifetime I had no trouble bouncing a basketball.

"I can't quite get a smooth rhythm," he continued. "The difference in the control is, when the ball comes up to my fingers (with the right hand), I can sense where it's at and put it right into the palms and press it back down again. The problem is, with the left hand, it's like it gets up there and it takes like a double dribble to get it down."

As usual, Kino's observations were remarkably astute.

I thought this difficulty represented residual of his hemineglect, such that he wasn't quite registering things with the affected left side (as occurred with the giveway weakness).

To my surprise, this session would prove to make a difference in these things…

CHAPTER EIGHTY-THREE

Subject: Qi Gong in the Treatment of TBI – 7th training session
Date: Wednesday, March 30, 2022 Minute 2
Safer driving…

Kino commented that sensation was particularly improved with his affected left hand.

"I have sustained a lot of the feeling," he said. "And I'm happy. I can feel so much more."

He talked about driving his older classic car and how it was that the improved sensation had been helpful for steering.

"So that I'm happy," he said. "I see that improvement. I feel safer about driving the car…."

CHAPTER EIGHTY-FOUR

Subject: Qi Gong in the Treatment of TBI – 7th training session
Date: Wednesday, March 30, 2022 Minute 15
"…come a long way…"

Kino turned his attention to the nunchuks.

"We've come a long way," he said, demonstrating not only circular movement ("helicopter") with nunchuks using his affected left hand, but also making a figure 8. "I'm able to do this now and keep talking and not even look at it. Just focus on other things."

He felt this improvement extended to the difficulties he'd been having at the shoulder.

"It used to require a lot of energy," he said. "Instead of just a flick of the wrist, I have to do a lot of control of my shoulder. It takes my whole arm working, so I get fatigued faster. But at least I'm able to do this without hitting my head now."

"So I'm happy to see the results," he concluded. "And as long as it takes, we're working on it…"

CHAPTER EIGHTY-FIVE

Subject: Qi Gong in the Treatment of TBI – 7th training session
Date: Wednesday, March 30, 2022 Minute 24
Neuropsychiatric assessment…

Kino was somber as he described his previous Neuropsychiatric assessment.

"I got a poor assessment," he said. "And then, I went there on the second round, and she advised me that some of the things that she may conclude could impact my life in such a way that I would not be able to return to work if they found something.

"And I said, 'OK, that's it. I'm done. I'm not going there.' Because I feel like I'm just fine. I don't want a doctor to tell me I can't work again.

"I have proven myself time and time again - Returning to work and accomplishing these great tasks of workload that we're dealing with currently."

And he had, I thought…

CHAPTER EIGHTY-SIX

Subject: Qi Gong in the Treatment of TBI – 7th training session
Date: Wednesday, March 30, 2022 Minute 26
"Electrifying…"

Testing Kino's sensation, it followed the usual pattern of improve sensation, with an electrical feeling for the digits of his left hand for light touch and pinprick

Of note, vibration sense appeared to be significantly improved, such that he did not describe much in the way of an electrical feeling, and just the sensation feeling equal between The fingers of his two hands.

Temperature also seemed improved, again without an 'electric' component…

CHAPTER EIGHTY-SEVEN

Subject: Qi Gong in the Treatment of TBI – 7th training session
Date: Wednesday, March 30, 2022 Minute 36

Kino demonstrated his use of the bouncing balloon. His rhythm was essentially equal between the two hands, and this he did with two balloons of different sizes and level of inflation (Though he did expressed some increased fatigue for the left shoulder)…

CHAPTER EIGHTY-EIGHT

Subject: Qi Gong in the Treatment of TBI – 7th training session
Date: Wednesday, March 30, 2022 Minute 44

Being that as well as recorded, the session was being photographed, I suggested we perform the tangibility exercise?

Kino immediately experienced a feeling of warmth over my hand. Indeed, he perceived so much energy from the point there, so as to ask me whether I was "hot"?

In addition, he noted a "tapering" quality to the energy, such that it diminished gradually.

"Yeah, there's a warmth," he said. "The whole hand. it's sort of just like glides or tapers… It never really goes away. It tapers to a less intense heat as I get towards the elbow. Very hot, very warm over your hand - Yes."

I noted that he'd been perceiving the energy with his right hand and was curious what he would perceive with the affected left hand?

In this case, he only perceived energy at one point in my palm (which he pinpointed to a crease there) and experienced none of the 'energy tapering' that he felt with the right.

"It's very warm over the crease," he said. "And that's it. There's no tapering effect."

In the act of repeating the exercise, Kino's system ultimately came to adjust, so that his perception of energy points became the same between his two hands.

"Thank you," he said. "We haven't done that before."

I wondered if this would help with the restoration of sensation in his affected left hand…

CHAPTER EIGHTY-NINE

Subject: Qi Gong in the Treatment of TBI – 7th training session
Date: Wednesday, March 30, 2022 Minute 48
"…a gentle ride…"

As Kino had described difficulties with the left shoulder, the Qi Gong treatment was initiated on his left side near shoulder, where energy vectors were immediately perceived.

"I don't know what you're messing with," Kino said, "but it feels like you're lifting my head up."

He described a feeling like I was "playing" with his left shoulder.

"I usually have crepitus in my left shoulder," he said, "and it feels like you lubricated the socket and made the crepitus feel less profound."

"Now, you're tugging my body to the left," he continued, "so that it's pulsating down. It feels like a gravitational pull. Like I had a bottle of tequila, and I'm stuck to the ground. But more like it's pulling me in that direction [He indicated to the left]. Like I'm totally drunk, with an 'I can't get up feeling.' Like the gravity is just pulling you. It's a gravitational type pull I'm feeling. It's like a wave or a throbbing function."

After following the energy to several feet away, now the energy was directing me back to where I'd begun at Kino's left shoulder.

Kino described the feeling like the "atmospheric pressure were decreasing… and my body was opening up. Like if I were to take a deep breath, it feels like I would take up more space. Like you were airing me out like a balloon, but from the outside."

Kino indicated this was a unique experience that he hadn't had before.

Meanwhile, the energy now had directed me to Kino's right side, at his head.

"Now it feels like you're moving around the ventricles of my brain," he said. "Like there's more fluid in the left occiput of my head, putting pressure on what I believe to be my own ear. A different type of pressure there."

"Now you're playing with the pressure behind my nasal sinus at my left," he continued.

When I inquired, he indicated he had not previously suffered from sinus problems.

"I have allergies, but I never got sinus infections," he said.

Again, he had not had feeling less like this before.

"It's a very strange feeling for the last several minutes," he commented. "It's like my brain was at the center of the old Atari joystick and playing Pac-Man," though adding that it had been "a gentle ride…"

CHAPTER NINETY

Subject: Qi Gong in the Treatment of TBI – 7th training session
Date: Wednesday, March 30, 2022 Minute 101
The end of hemineglect…

The energy evaporated from my hands - though it still felt as though I were interfacing with it, as there was a sensation of expansion in my head. It felt like my cranial fissures had opened, facilitating a very pleasant feeling in my skull.

Kino, too, described the session as "different."

"I feel like I have water in my head," he said. "From the cerebellum area, parietal and just a little at the frontal on the left side. Why I don't know? My injured side is here [He indicated the right side]."

I asked if we could reevaluate him?

First, I examined the sensation in his own fingers.

"Even the soft touch is pretty well equal," he said.

He commented that he was experiencing a sensation of energy at his middle finger.

"And that is significantly different!" he declared, forcefully. "The soft touch practically feels the same!"

This pattern continued for pinprick and vibration sense.

He appeared somewhat tentative for coordination testing with finger to nose and rapid alternating movements, but improved.

Kino inquired if his reflexes could be evaluated, saying, "I'd like to focus on my reflexes, because I'd like to ride the motorcycle… and I don't want to wreck it."

There was persistent hyperreflexia on the left side.

However, to my surprise, when I evaluate him for strength testing, there wasn't a giveaway weakness on the left side this time!

This represented a remarkable improvement; it was as though he'd overcome his issues of hemineglect!

"Do you think there's a difference?" he asked, doubtful.

I responded in the affirmative.

"Thank you for that," he responded, moved. "I don't get to test things besides the therapy we're doing now to learn what things I can do to reinforce that…"

CHAPTER NINETY-ONE

Subject: Qi Gong in the Treatment of TBI – 7th training session
Date: Wednesday, March 30, 2022 Minute 114

Kino went to the bouncing balloon: Wrist flexion was still slower on the left side; however, it was still improved.

He demonstrated with the nunchuks: Again, there was some progress with his wrist movement on the left, especially when transitioning from the circular (helicopter) movement to figure 8.

"I would've beat myself up with it before," he commented.

Then, he went to dribbling the basketball and was quick to not the gains he had sustained.

"This is improved from what I did earlier," he said.

Indeed, he was cupping the ball with his left hand, whereas he had not done that before the Qi Gong treatment.

"That was improvement," he repeated. "Thank you, doctor…"

CHAPTER NINETY-TWO

Subject: Qi Gong in the Treatment of TBI – 8th training session
Date: Wednesday, April 6, 2022 Minute 0

Kino began his 8th Qi Gong training session by demonstrating his dribbling of the basketball.

"I'm doing better than I did it last week," he said.

I agreed. Like at the end of the session last week, he was again cupping the ball with his left hand and meeting it with each dribble.

"I think there's a lot of improvement with the numbness sensation, too," he declared.

On neurologic evaluation, sensation between the two hands was essentially the same. Again, the main difference was an "electrical sensation" that he experienced with stimuli to the digits of the left hand.

Strength testing confirmed the retention of improved strength, such that give way weakness was no longer present!

Kino demonstrated improved nunchuk ability, with the left shoulder more open and with more movement. Bouncing balloon was the same.

Reflexes were still hyperreflexic on the left and there was still some slowness on finger to nose; however, rapid alternating movements were decidedly improved, with much improve speed that Kino thought was attributable to the increased mobility in his left shoulder.

"It's like it was stuck before," he said of his shoulder. "Compared to now, when I went with it and focused on letting it go."

Kino commented that he appreciated that both Bill and I were both present today to perform Qi Gong during this session.

"Not to downplay the help last week, but I feel like I notice more of a difference the weeks that Bill and you are both doing it," he said.

"It's like we complement each other," Bill offered.

I agreed with Bill. Indeed, later when Bill and I would perform the Qi Gong self-practice together, it would become apparent that whereas I was more connected with the heavens, he was more connected with the earth.

"It's like you [Bill] can take the Chi you've never seen, absorb it," Kino asserted. "And then Dr. Yanuck takes the leftover Chi, absorbs it, and he doesn't have much space in his Chi, because he has a full tank from pulling that Chi out of people."

Nevertheless, Bill was impressed with Kino's progress and offered the following assessment.

"I saw a lot of improvement in you this time," Bill said, so to suggest Kino had benefited significantly from the last treatment despite Bill having not been present…

CHAPTER NINETY-THREE

Subject: Qi Gong in the Treatment of TBI – 8th training session
Date: Wednesday, April 6, 2022 Minute 20

The Qi Gong treatment began, I was surprised to find a very definite energy factor coming from Kino,

"Like maybe we have gone through a lot of chaotic, subtle energy, and now we're getting to more specific stuff?" I postulated.

In the act of reevaluating Kino, Bill pursued the energy further than I'd ever seen him do so before, following the energy out some two or three feet from Kino's body.

"I could feel it clearly out that far," Bill asserted. "Before it kind of dissipated."

Furthermore, he had developed a feeling for directionality with the energy disturbances.

"Yes, I do," he responded…

CHAPTER NINETY-FOUR

Subject: Qi Gong in the Treatment of TBI – 8th training session
Date: Wednesday, April 6, 2022 Minute 24

Kino described feeling something of a "gravitational pull to the left."

"One thing I notice about Bill," Kino said. "I don't know how close you guys are getting, but there's always a warmth that I can sense before, after and during."

"I don't know how close he's getting to my body," Kino added, "but I can always feel the warmth."

Kino added that he didn't experience that 'warmth' when I worked with him.

"There is a difference between the two of you," he asserted.

I wondered that that wouldn't change, now that Bill was getting more comfortable pursuing energy disturbances further from the body…

CHAPTER NINETY-FIVE

Subject: Qi Gong in the Treatment of TBI – 8th training session
Date: Wednesday, April 6, 2022 Minute 27

"I can still feel that gravitational pull," Kino said. "It's like a shifting of fluid inside my head. Makes me wonder, Am I wobbly?"

I'd been following an energy strain on his left.

"It's like my neck has been gravitationally pulled towards you," he continued. "Towards the doorway."

I went back and checked for residual energy strains.

"It's like I feel something in the rotator cuff," he said.

I wondered if the back of the examination table should be elevated, so to support him should the joint want to move?

"Yeah, I saw you jumping around like a fish," he responded. "Let's see what happens."

I scanned over the area again: With my right hand at his shoulder, I found the energy dimmed when my left hand got to the area around Kino's brow (at the third eye chakra).

I shared this with Bill, and he found the same.

I went back, located the energy Kino's third eye chakra and then follow the energy's path. It quickly took me all the way across the room.

I invited Bill to go back and scan over Kino.

"It's much smaller," he said of the energy coming off the left shoulder. "Almost like it's not there anymore. And not over his head also."

I discussed the importance of the third eye chakra.

"That's the place right between the chakras you rely on for living in the world, and the crown chakra, which connects you with the universal ideals. It's right between heaven and earth. Right between contending with issues of survival, and contending with the higher ideals, like altruism, sacrifice and spirituality.

"So, it's not surprising to find that people who have experienced trauma now have significant chakra imbalances at the third eye."

As I worked to release the strain, I inquired have Kino as doing?

"Resting," he responded. "Feeling really comfortable."

Bill left the room, and I continued working.

The energy directed me back to Kino.

Then, the energy took to having 'in-and-out' movement, not unlike breathing.

I shared that chakra adjustments could often be significant – so to create significant energetic realignment within the body and have profound results compared to other energy disturbances.

Kino reiterated his experiences with the Neuropsych testing, especially as regarded the threat that "if they read something, it could mean that I possibly won't be able to work again."

I wondered if that experience was traumatizing to Kino? After all, Kino treated the ability to work like his ability to live in the world. He'd said as much previously. At the same time, I was certain his rational mind was probably telling him to work with his doctors. Perhaps this was why we were finding this chakra disturbance at the third eye?

He described his experience observing the court proceedings involving his assailant.

"I watched the guy get put in prison who did this to me," he said. "I watched every court case on zoom. And strangely, it's bothering me recently because the location where I was attacked is the same exact area that was described in the Sacramento mass shooting business."

The shooting occurred at around 2:00 a.m. in the area of 10th Street and K Street, just blocks away from the California State Capitol. There were six fatalities in the shooting: three men and three women. Another 12 people suffered from varying degrees of injury. Four were taken to the trauma unit at UC Davis Medical Center, where Kino had been taken when he suffered his TBI.

"On 10th St. near L," Kino said. "Does that area just have a thing for injuring people? I don't know if that's going to spark some kind of PTSD. I'm a responsible gun owner. I don't want my weapons taken away."

He talked about another VA employee and gun owner who lost his rights to possess weapons.

"I'm a hunter," he continued. "I'm a sports rifleman. And most importantly, I want to be protected. It would end my life if this ever happened again."

The energy coming from Kino was taking my hands towards the ceiling.

"I haven't been down there and walked that area of Sacramento since that night," he said. "And I don't want to go back there. I'm not going back there."

Kino indicated that he was feeling tension in the back of his neck, as well as a headache.

"Right smack in the middle between the top and the bottom on the right side in the back of my head," he said.

This was around the area of his traumatic brain injury.

"There's definitely tension in my neck, and there shouldn't be, because I'm just sitting here with my body rested," Kino said.

I was working with very subtle energy in the ether level.

"It feels like you're messing with my fake skull," Kino said, referring to the prosthetic skull that had been placed some months after his traumatic brain injury.

"I'm getting a strange, numb, tingly feeling in my left middle finger," Kino continued.

This, of course, with the place of Kino's greatest sensory difficulties.

Following the energy, I invited Bill to go back and see if there was a difference?

"This is almost gone," Bill commented of the energy over Kino's right side.

"I don't feel the warmth of Bill like I did on the left side," Kino commented. "Not on the right side. I hear his voice and I know he's over there."

I wondered what that could be? Why he wouldn't perceive Bill on that right side?

"Maybe energy can't pass through the prosthetic?" Kino offered.

I went back to Kino's left side and pursued an energy path from there; then, I invited Bill to check over there.

"There's still warm on the left," Kino commented.

Bill followed the energy of a long way off from Kino, which was quite different from his usual pattern of following the energy three-dimensionally, rather than two-dimensionally the way I had?

"Yeah," Bill affirmed of his performing the practice two-dimensionally. "Almost like pulling it like a string."

Then, Bill encountered a new phenomenon that he hadn't been privy to before.

"It's interesting," he commented. "I'm trying to figure out where it's going. Because it's coming and moving around in circles."

He indicated that the circular movement was in the counterclockwise direction.

As it happened, I loved to immerse myself in energy vertices and happily pursued the energy disturbance that Bill described.

It took me in a counter clockwise circle that was relatively short-lived, so that I quickly invited Bill to go back and see what he observed this time.

"It's gone now," he said. "I don't feel it. Last time when I was about here, it was warm, and now it's gone."

The energy was holding in place, so that as much as I wanted to get back and continue scanning Kino, I was not able, and wondered if this was telling me that I was finished for now, and how the others felt, and whether they also felt like we had done enough for today, or wanted to continue?

"No, I got a bit of a peace, like I'm done, too," Kino declared.

Re-evaluating Kino for changes like extension of the fingers of his left hand, he seemed moved by the improvements.

"We've come so far since doing this," Kino said, affected.

Kino wanted to test himself with a sharper object to evaluate his sensation, particularly in the middle finger.

"There's the electrical feeling," he said, of the left digit.

Then, comparing the feeling between the two sides, he commented, "Very similar. More similar than what they were before."

Coordination for finger to nose was improved for the left side, with less hesitation, and rapid alternating movements was so much better and faster!

The bouncing balloon was improved for his left side, and his wrist action improved.

"There's more reflex in my hand compared to before," Kino affirmed.

But he looked tired, and added disparagingly, "I put more stress in my shoulder."

Kino shook his head and slumped to shoulders, as though discouraged over his improvements.

He's asking for so much! I thought. This was so different from me, who's typically delighted with the least incremental progress!

I conveyed that he'd displayed significantly more mobility and ease and openness at the left shoulder than there'd been in the beginning of the session, such that there was significant improvement.

Bill affirmed this.

"I'm also seeing a lot of improvement," he said. "I wasn't here the last time, but from the session before that until now, I'm seeing a lot of improvement."

Still, Kino appeared discouraged, as he looked down at his affected left hand.

"I've got to challenge myself physically," he asserted.

He'd brought a softball, and picked it up now and instructed me to throw it at him.

"Like throw this right at my face," he demanded, "to get me to wave it off."

I did as he asked; with his affected left hand, he batted the ball away.

"That's the threat," he insisted. "Block a punch coming at me."

I nodded, as I now understood: The reason his improvements weren't good enough for him... The reason he was pushing so hard to regain his abilities, was because (for him) it was a matter of survival…

CHAPTER NINETY-SIX

Subject: Qi Gong in the Treatment of TBI – 8th training session
Date: Wednesday, April 6, 2022 Minute 1:09

If health is the name for life when it is flourishing, then the healing force is the same as the life-force, and comes from the whole - not from surgical or chemical intervention.
~ Paulos Mar Gregorios, Healing – A Holistic Approach

He went to dribbling the basketball. Again, there was better cupping of the ball and anticipating it with his left hand, so to appear more natural and coordinated, and I reminded him of how far he'd come.

"I'm hopeful," he responded. "I'm never going to give up on this. I'm never going to give up. I know that through will… I'm never going to give up.

"And I thank you for your help. It's like, that's why I keep coming. I see it, as well.

"I love hearing the feedback. This is kind of why I'm grateful that I'm in the medical field."

"This is amazing," he concluded. "It's not a pill. It's not surgery. It's just exciting to see this stuff."

He had no idea how exciting it was for me…

CHAPTER NINETY-SEVEN

In spite of all the advances by Kino, events would lead me to have to get back to the original objectives of the project; that being, the application of Qi Gong to treat problems of addiction.

It came about this way: Representatives from the Innovation Accelerator Program reached out, saying, "We are looking into some possible options for you to be highly successful in spreading this further than Mather. Please give me a call when you are free so we can see what type of flexibility there is with a few alternative options."

They inquired about developing a possible video series for people to learn online prior to in-person training. And they were particularly interested in the thoughts of our subject matter expert, Dr. K, since she'd been consistently following the project online and whether that had prepared her for the planned in-person training next month.

So, I reached out to Dr. K, sure that I'd receive a positive response.

What I got, instead, was the following:

Hi Mike!

I figured we might be able to discuss this in person but happy to start the dialogue as it pertains to my personal experience:

1. I think it can be helpful to watch a few sessions but candidly I'm not sure how much I am getting out of watching it week per week outside of seeing his progress. Which is great but I'm not sure how this is helping me learn to do it myself. I understand that energy work can be beneficial so don't feel I need this "proof of concept".

2. Having more hands-on experiences would be helpful. I think you mentioned that Qi Gong is traditionally practiced by the individual as opposed to the model that you are teaching us. Maybe we can learn how to do the individual work (not sure how long this takes) so that we can start practice working with energy?

3. I noticed that we have not worked with someone with an SUD [Substance Use Disorder] and am wondering how this might apply to my patient population?

4. I will honestly not be seeing my patients in person. So one question I have had is, can this be taught to be virtually so that I can then help my veterans virtually?

Does that help? What are your thoughts?

Best, Dr. K…

'What are your thoughts?' I re-read, rhetorically, as I stared helplessly into the computer monitor. *I'm doomed!*

She wants 'Virtual Qi Gong.' And I've got all of three weeks to develop that practice and teach her before she flies down here for in-person training!

It's not like I hadn't taught it before; but recently I'd received feedback that put me on edge.

Let me explain…

CHAPTER NINETY-EIGHT

When I came to the VA Research Department with my interest in studying Qi Gong, they paired me with a 'scientific mentor' (who I'll refer to as Prof. P) to advise me when it came to putting together a proposal.

Shortly thereafter, Prof. P confided that among the reasons she was interested in the assignment was because she had a childhood friend who (from the time he was a teenager) had a talent for "energy harvesting and reading accurately the sources of people's health and related problems, but tells me that he lost it over time."

"I do not think he has had any formal training in these things," she continued. "I let him borrow your book, and now he is interested in meeting you and talking to you."

I'll refer to my mentor's friend as B. Talking with him, he described a childhood filled with horrific physical and mental abuse, from which he was still suffering.

It happened that B only lived about a hundred miles away, so I suggested we meet in-person.

But he requested that we attempt a 'remote' healing session, saying that he just had a feeling that remote healing would help him.

Feeling it couldn't do any harm, I agreed and focused on him and his life story and opened myself to any energy I might be sensing. In time, energy filled my hands as I followed it in the directions that it took them. Then, some minutes later, I experienced a feeling of energy at my head, as though tethering me between the crown chakra and the universe, and kindling the memory of an experience I'd had some twenty-five years before. It happened this way...

I'd been caring for my first love's mother, employing bioenergy and Qi Gong. When my work was done and it was time to leave the family, I was expecting it to be as difficult (as it always was because I loved them so much). Hence, stepping onto a departing Greyhound bus and taking a seat in the back, I drew a deep breath and wondered, 'When is it going to hit? The remorse and sadness?'

However, as the bus drove off, as opposed to the familiar emptiness and hollowness in my chest, I experienced a sensation of energy. Starting at my head, the energy filled me, till beaming and overflowing to every part of me, so that it felt like I was enveloped in a cocoon of energy, fuller and more expansive than anything I'd ever experienced before!

'I've honored something,' were the words that came to me. 'I've shown some great respect. It's something simple, yet wonderful. It reaches to the core of my being – God is love...'

And that's what I was feeling now as I worked with B remotely, leading me to believe that (more than anything else) what B needed to facilitate his healing was to release the retained energy of trauma associated with troubled, trauma filled world of his childhood by tapping into and connecting with the universal energy of love…

CHAPTER NINETY-NINE

As B and I continued these remote healing sessions, the experience was more and more profound: I entered a state of profound relaxation, as the retained energy of trauma locked everywhere in my body (muscles, tendons, ligaments, etc.) left me, as though having boarded some conveyor belt to the heavens, being pulled up by an energy sink in the sky.

"Yeah, while you stay grounded, the energy can move up," B agreed.

Indeed, all fatigue and weariness left me during these sessions, replaced by a feeling of profound rejuvenation.

Nevertheless, even B's good friend, Prof. P, questioned the plausibility of these remote healing sessions.

"That suggests that the bioenergy experience is psychological rather than physical," she asserted.

To this I responded that obviously I can't explain this phenomenon on any known physiologic terms; however, there's a lot we don't know about this field, so I'm not ready to exclude the possibility of connecting energetically over a distance.

For example, back at the start of the Internet, I would have never imagined using it without my computer attached to an ethernet cable – Now, we take wireless connections for granted.

So, can the energies flow between people over significant distances? Who knows? Maybe it's like getting the Internet without a cable?

"Because Chi works on a purely energetic level," one Qi Gong healer commented, "the distance between the practitioner and the client is not a limiting factor, as energy is not restricted by space or

time. In fact, certain people respond better to distant healing treatments than to in-person sessions…"

So, the groundwork had been laid down for performing Qi Gong virtually.

Now, I had to develop a step-by-step format for it…

CHAPTER ONE HUNDRED

Ball of Energy exercise

First, I'd seen where some had trained in energy perception via the 'Ball of Energy' exercise: Seated comfortably, place your hands (palms facing each other) about 6 inches apart and imagine that you are holding an energy ball between them. See if you don't perceive some energy at your palms, either in the form of heat or static electricity or tingling at your fingertips or coolness or throbbing or puffs of air or a breeze or feeling of 'magnetic' attraction or repulsion. Next, move your palms together and then farther apart to get a sense of the energy ball (or bubble). I figured I'd attempt to make this the first step in the virtual practice…

CHAPTER ONE HUNDRED AND ONE

Crown Chakra activation

Next, I'd move to Crown Chakra activation.

Based on my work with Mr. B, I'd suggest gradually allowing the hands to move apart in an arcing fashion till they came to rest (palms up) on one's sides, while still perceiving the energy in the hands. Then, raising the hands slowly (shoulder length apart) upwards. It was my experience that when my hands were at about the level of my heart, it would activate a feeling of energy at my head, so to suggest the opening of the crown chakra, thereby connecting the trainee with the Universal Qi, with the theoretical capacity to reconcile all forms of trauma and optimally restore body function (Gong).

With the crown chakra now activated, I would instruct the lowering of the hands back to the sides then sitting comfortably experiencing the energy radiating upwards from the hands and crown chakra, allowing the retained energy of trauma to leave the body and flow outwards into the Ethosphere, leaving the body feeling less tense and more relaxed.

Then, to sit with this way for several minutes until the feeling of energy at your hands and head dissipates, signaling the release of retained energy of trauma to the extent that the body desired.

So, I'd developed a form of virtual Qi Gong practice, mostly based on my real-life experience.

Now, I'd attempt it with Dr. K...

CHAPTER ONE HUNDRED AND TWO

What follows are the notes from the first Qi Gong self-practice training session with Dr. K. I'll try not to make them too 'clinical.' Of note, this and all the other Qi Gong sessions were recorded.

As well as Dr. K and myself, the Addiction Recovery Treatment Services (ARTS) Nurse Care Manager, Bill was present (though he arrived late).

Unlike the other books about this project, I'm going to share more of my thoughts and comments during the session – This because Dr. K asked a number of questions that touched on Qi Gong theory. Hence, in contrast to my usual pattern in these books about the project (of keeping my voice to a minimum in these works, so to keep the focus on those navigating the Qi Gong experience for the first time), I'm going to share.

As usual, for those of you interested in learning more about my experience in this area, I'll refer you to my book, Bioenergy Therapy.

Getting back to the Qi Gong self-practice training that follows, I'm going to endeavor to share it in simple, clear and concise language in the hope that that will make these sessions easier to follow.

Subject: Qi Gong Self-Practice - Training 1
Date: Wednesday, April 13, 2022 Minute 0
"...a feeling of pulling..."

Beginning with the ball of energy exercise, Dr. K quickly lifted a brow.

"I have a feeling of pulling," she said. "I don't know if that is energy?... It's at the meatier part of the hand."

Previously, Dr. K had indicated that she'd had some experience with energy medicine. Now I inquired if she'd had some perception of energy?

"So, I worked with an energy healer," she began, "she'd talk about 'pulses', like energy pulses, and she tried to get me to feel them, and I couldn't."

"But I went to a workshop with her," she added, "and I could feel some things. A sense of energy moving, yes."

I asked if what she was feeling now compared to that?

She indicated in the affirmative.

"Mmm hmmm," she said.

I suggested she attempt to move her hands apart, while maintaining the perception of energy.

"How far do I have to go before I lose it?" she asked.

I indicated that the intent was not to "lose it", but move the hands apart with some perception of energy still there.

"Initially when I pulled my hands apart, it just went to nothing, like I couldn't feel anything," she responded. "But, thinking about it more consciously, it feels like the space is being filled the more I go apart – as opposed to feeling a smaller ball of energy that I'm getting further away from."

At this point, Bill joined us for the self-practice session. Dr. K and I took a break, as I helped Bill set up the computer in the other room, so to join us virtually from there…

CHAPTER ONE HUNDRED AND THREE

Subject: Qi Gong Self-Practice - Training 1
Date: Wednesday, April 13, 2022 Minute 7
Drag…

Returning to Dr. K, we re-initiated the self-practice, starting with the ball of energy and then moving her hands apart.

"So, you're saying that I should feel it even though my hands are not holding the ball of energy?" she asked.

I demonstrated it myself, holding the ball of energy, and then moving my hands apart (the energy still in my hands), until they were comfortably on my lap, palms up.

"OK, I can try it," she said.

Then she stopped.

"That's interesting," she said. "My hands were resting on my keyboard, and when I moved back, I sort of lost it, so I'm going to have to start over."

Yes, changes in tactile sensation often affected energy perception, so to have to "Start over."

The session was again interrupted because of Bill difficulties that Bill was having with the computer in the other room.

Nevertheless, although not intended, this and the other interruption might have had benefitted Dr. K by giving her more practice with the approach. Indeed, each time, Dr. K found that she could move through the different parts of the exercise quicker.

"I think I got to it faster," she commented…

CHAPTER ONE HUNDRED AND FOUR

Subject: Qi Gong Self-Practice - Training 1
Date: Wednesday, April 13, 2022 Minute 15
"...lifting the ball of energy..."

Next, I instructed Dr. K in the crown chakra activation part of the self-practice, instructing her to lift her hands so too activate the crown chakra.

"Are we lifting the ball of energy up?" she asked. "Or are we just moving our hands?"

I explained that, for whatever reason, the process occurred best when there was energy perception in the hands. Then, as the hands moved upwards, it just seemed that the crown chakra opened.

"OK, I can feel it at the top of my head," she indicated. "It's not like at the tip top of my head, but at a 45° angle."

Dr. K described the feeling of energy.

"I could feel tingling," she said. "Starting at my forehead and then going up. And now it feels kind of like my hands are. It feels like there's a band like my headphones, but not my headphones, and I think that's because that's where my hands are, and it feels concentrated. Like maybe that's because that's where my hands are positioned. Yeah."

Her hands were above the level of her shoulders, and I wondered that Dr. K wasn't defining the boundaries of the energy being released at her crown chakra?...

CHAPTER ONE HUNDRED AND FIVE

Subject: Qi Gong Self-Practice - Training 1
Date: Wednesday, April 13, 2022 Minute 18

As the self-practice progressed, Dr. K inquired what I was feeling? I responded that I was feeling immersed in a feeling of energy all around me that was accompanied by a feeling of awe and reverence that typically accompanies connecting energetically while working directly with patients or the Universal Chi.

"It's definitely a pleasant feeling," she commented. "Since moving my hands around, it feels like the parts of my head that I'm getting the sensation are contingent on where my hand placement is."

"And it feels really calm," she added. "It feels nice."

I shared the Chi Gong teaching that the energy at the head/crown chakra facilitated a connection with the 'Universal Chi', this theoretical blueprint for all life that had the capacity to help reconcile any form of trauma. This could be regarded as something of the 'great computer in the sky', that we could sync with and could help correct and reboot any 'damaged program' in our system…

CHAPTER ONE HUNDRED AND SIX

Subject: Qi Gong Self-Practice - Training 1
Date: Wednesday, April 13, 2022 Minute 22

Dr. K appeared to be appreciating following the energy with her hands, so I let her go with it.

I pondered the question of how 'in touch' she was with her innate intelligence? Could she let the Qi guide her, as it had with me that time with Sam when I made that breakthrough with Qi emission? Such as that was considered 'very advanced' where the practice of Qi Gong was concerned, and not something expected of a beginner (to say nothing of someone entirely new to the practice like Dr. K was).

But at the time that I began my practice of Qi Gong, I'd been considered 'advanced', too – This primarily because of my training in Bioenergy. And Dr. K had shared that she worked with an 'energy healer', as well as described being something of a devout member of a Buddhist temple.

So, I couldn't be sure how much experience and innate abilities Dr. K was bringing to the practice, but it seemed to me they could be considerable…

CHAPTER ONE HUNDRED AND SEVEN

Subject: Qi Gong Self-Practice - Training 1
Date: Wednesday, April 13, 2022 Minute 25

Dr. K raised the question of 'intention' in this approach?

"I feel like with energy work," she began, "a lot of the times, there's talk of intention. Are we setting intentions when we start our practice? Like do we say, 'Our hope is to release trauma?' Or do we say anything? Or have any intention in mind? Or is it more passive?"

Yes. In my previous Energy Medicine support groups, I structured the class so that we would first work with new members, while the 'regulars' offered their attention and intention to that person, so to direct more healing energy towards the person.

At the same time, though, I did not want my intentions to overwhelm my ability to be in tune with the patient's energetic circulation.

For example, when it came to Kino, I was endlessly fascinated with the restoration of sensation that he was undergoing (after having diminished sensation for so many years following his TBI), so that I could not wait to get back to working with him again in that area.

But at the same time, I was open to the possibility that his body-mind might be saying, 'Hey, I appreciate that you really want to get to this, but there's something else more important to me.'

I noted that in the last session with Kino, it was interesting that Bill and I found that blockage in his third eye had to be released before we could release the retained energy of trauma in his affected left hand.

All this was a long way of saying it was important to approach healing with enthusiasm and interest and intention (and even specific

desires to facilitate improvement for the other person); but at the same time be open to the possibility that the body-mind might have its own agenda as to what it needed most and what it needed first, so to facilitate healing.

Because in this form of healing, I held that the central tenet was to give the body what it needed, when it needed it, where it needed it, at the exact dose required, and not be forceful…

CHAPTER ONE HUNDRED AND EIGHT

Subject: Qi Gong Self-Practice - Training 1
Date: Wednesday, April 13, 2022 Minute 28

Dr. K inquired about the amount of time needed for the self-practice? I responded that I didn't have a set amount of time that I suggested, and that usually I practiced for as long as I felt immersed in the feeling of energy.

I added that I thought a few minutes would do, but then considered how it was that I was continuously surprised at the length of time that Bill and I would work with Kino, as they were usually hour-long sessions, which was considerably longer than the few minutes that I usually performed bioenergy with someone?

I wondered that that mostly came from the interplay between Bill and Kino and myself, and the benefit that working in a group offers within this approach.

Indeed, as well as the sessions being longer than usual, the results with Kino have been more striking than anyone else I had ever worked with in my 30-years' experience with this approach and really beyond my wildest expectations for the project.

I mean, we were watching him undergo the restoration of neurologic function after years of neurologic deficits! What could be more exciting?…

CHAPTER ONE HUNDRED AND NINE

Subject: Qi Gong Self-Practice - Training 1
Date: Wednesday, April 13, 2022 Minute 29

I shared with Dr. K that it was interesting it seemed the focus of my self-practice was facilitating breathing, as my hands were going in and out, as though to pattern themselves after the expanding and contracting of my lungs and chest wall.

Indeed, over the course of these sessions, it was becoming easier for me to breathe. In addition, my chest was literally expanding, so that I could no longer fit into my white dress shirts!

Meanwhile, I inquired how she was doing?

"Yeah, good," she said. "It feels like a big ball of energy."

I inquired if she was still perceiving something at her crown chakra?

"Mmm hmmm," she acknowledged.

I asked if she felt this was an adequate self-practice for introducing it to those new to Qi Gong who were interested in learning it virtually?

"I think it's a great idea," she responded. "Originally, just thinking about our progress so far, I think the first several sessions, and seeing you all work, there was a general sense of, 'What's going on?' - seeing your movements and also listening to you all speak to each other and us. But I think that a practical component [of virtual self-practice], then if you have that, that's really helpful.

"Because the thing is, as I've said to you, my folks are virtual, and I'm committing to this because I want to learn how to do it, but really it's going to be something that I'll probably only offer virtually. So, I think being able to be taught in that modality, Well… You asked me to, 'try to get somebody that you can work on, and I'll guide you…' But, ultimately, learning if this can be done in virtual space (and I know that you have done it in a virtual space), that's where I'm coming from."

Then, she stopped speaking, abruptly.

"And I think I lost my ball of energy," she said, smiling and laughing…

CHAPTER ONE HUNDRED AND TEN

Subject: Qi Gong Self-Practice - Training 1
Date: Wednesday, April 13, 2022 Minute 35

Bill had got the computer going in the other room, so that now all three of us could attempt this virtually from different locations.

First, I took Bill through the ball of energy exercise.

"Try to spread your hands apart and maintain that energy perception," I said. "Do this in an arcing fashion, so that your hands ultimately come to rest at your sides, palms up."

Then I directed everyone to move their hands upwards until there was an awareness for energy at the crown chakra.

"Yeah, I'm finding spots," he acknowledged.

It was, in general, Bill's tendency to scan with his hands very close to the body, and I explained that in the self-practice it was not so much meant to bring his hands to the head to perceive energy, as much of a matter of the energy 'turning on' at the crown chakra; i.e., the crown chakra being 'activated' at a certain point when the hands were raised, such that that was what triggered a feeling of energy at the head.

But like Dr. K had been, Bill was still focused on perceiving the energy at his head with his hands.

"I'm feeling it more in my hands," he admitted.

I decided to go with that, and inquired what he was feeling in his hands?

"Kind of a warmth," he said.

I inquired whether it had any directionality? And whether it took his hands anywhere? Bill took his time before responding.

"Up," he said.

Perfect, I thought.
Then, I explained…

CHAPTER ONE HUNDRED AND ELEVEN

Subject: Qi Gong Self-Practice - Training 1
Date: Wednesday, April 13, 2022 Minute 41

Qi Gong teaches that within the universal Chi was the blueprint for healing all things, so that if you could connect with that, it would help scan your system, looking for internal problems that resulted from trauma, and release the retained energy of trauma that stemmed from that. It was not unlike activating a computer malware program, so to perform an internal scan of the body, looking for and identifying damaged and corrupted programs, then repairing those programs, so to make them as optimally function as possible again.

And when you did this, and those programs were corrected, then your system would stop just spinning its wheels and going around and around trying to work and not being able to, wasting a lot of energy being stuck and held in place, such that that useless, retained energy could be released from the system. It was that retained energy of trauma that was leaving through our hands and crown chakra now.

As for myself, I could perform the self-practice for hours, and just feel my system relax and relax and relax, as that retained energy of trauma left me through the crown chakra, while maintaining the connection with the universal Chi that was just working on fixing more and more 'damaged programs' in my system, so to effect an input-output circuit of healing energy coming in and retained energy of trauma going out: The energy of healing from the universal Chi entering my system through the crown chakra and my hands to facilitate healing and repair; and the outpouring of retained energy of trauma out of my system as it left me.

And although this was like a meditation, the only thought in my head was being aware of this energy immersion and how pleasant that was.

In truth, it wasn't all that different from the feeling I got when I connected with the energetic circulation of someone else - Something that I experience with each and every person I work with this way, every time I apply this approach. How it was that whenever I connect with another's energetic circulation, I experienced a feeling of awe and reverence, such that I wanted to understand the other person suffering better, delve deeper, essentially serve as a better and more caring provider and healer to that person.

In this self-practice approach, that awe and reverence that I feel is for the universe.

I shared my "God is love" experience, about the first time this happened, in which on a bus ride home after caring for my first love's mother, rather than being filled with my usual feelings of sadness and remorse at leaving them, instead I was pleasantly immersed in this cocoon of energy (more than anything I had ever been experienced before), so to be so extraordinary to me that it left me to conclude, "God is love."

I described how it was that I usually kept my chest sunken, but when I practice the Qi Gong self-practice, my chest wanted to open, so to breathe and use my body more optimally, that, in turn, more comfortable and more free.

I said that I delighted in this experience and it happened best when I performed the self-practice in the company of others, including virtually…

CHAPTER ONE HUNDRED AND TWELVE

Subject: Qi Gong Self-Practice - Training 1
Date: Wednesday, April 13, 2022 Minute 47.

I inquired what Bill was experiencing?

"It's almost like a meditation," he responded. "I'm remembering when I participated in one of our groups a long time ago. It was a group in arts that was kind of a meditation kind of group, and it was about just kind of relaxing all of the muscles in your body, focusing on different areas... 'Mindfulness" is the skill... And I kind of got there because I was following the energy and I just kind of noticed my body."

He smiled and laughed.

This would mark the beginning of Bill using his newly acquired expertise in energy healing to take his training in meditation to places he had never taken it before.

Basically, his familiarity with mindfulness and his newfound skill in Qi Gong catalyzed his putting it all together, so to make meditation come alive and useful to him like it had never been before.

It was the energy 'piece' that he been missing. Now that he had that piece, he could take meditative practices to a whole new realm.

And, fortunately for us, he'd take us there, too...

CHAPTER ONE HUNDRED AND THIRTEEN

Subject: Qi Gong Self-Practice - Training 1
Date: Wednesday, April 13, 2022 Minute 48

I shared the comment from master chow suggesting that the Qi Gong master helps facilitate the Chi field, so to suggest that there might be something to people connecting this way and that our energies were interacting.

This led to the question: How is this possible? Dr. K is hundreds of miles away?

To that, I said I had no good explanation. But I wasn't willing to deny the possibility, either.

"Maybe it is possible and one day we'll learn how it is that when it comes to energy and there is a way to be simultaneously connected?" I said.

This, in turn, suggested the possibility that even beyond helping a person to connect with the universal Chi, that additionally it might be that your energies were interacting to help each other heal from energy disturbances that resulted from trauma, so to help each other release retained energy of trauma…

CHAPTER ONE HUNDRED AND FOURTEEN

Subject: Qi Gong Self-Practice - Training 1
Date: Wednesday, April 13 2022 Minute 50

Dr. K asked about specifics.

"How long do you typically sit for?" she asked. "Do you do it for as long as you can feel the energy? And then it just depends day-to-day?"

Yes, I responded, I would say that that was exactly right.

I described my experience with Master Chou: How it was that the first 90 days were about a series of bows and then standing while attempting to connect with a universal chi (as well as other things, like not engaging in sex and maintaining a vegan diet). Those 90 days felt like a long time and I couldn't say that I particularly enjoyed them or benefited from them.

So, how long was needed to do this initially before someone is ready to get more advanced training, I didn't know.

"Obviously, I didn't do this at all with Bill," I said, "and yet he was up and ready to go immediately when it came to working with Kino."

Dr. K commented that in the two times that we had performed the self-practice during this training, each time she stayed with the energy for about 15 minutes.

"I think that's how long it lasted for me both times," she said. "Bill, did you experience the same? I feel like it was 15 or 20 minutes, and then I sort of lost it. Did it feel like that for you? Or are you still feeling it?"

"Yeah," he responded. "I was following the energy, and then I kind of got distracted by a meditation, and I just wanted to follow that because it was very relaxing."

I asserted that I thought he had done the right thing, And to do what the body wanted while performing the self practice.

"Do what's healing," I declared. "This is not meant to be forceful. This is meant to be really fluid. You never know what kind of dose of this you need. A few minutes? A few seconds? Whatever. If that's what your body is telling you, and that's the sense you get, then go with it. Don't treat this like you have to push yourself to do it."

"As far as I'm concerned," I added, "if your mind goes somewhere else, let it go somewhere else. It's OK. Don't force it, or say, 'Oh, darn.' In my opinion, it takes practice."

There shouldn't be any harshness or judgment involved, I asserted. It might be important for you to integrate things along the way – like bringing the energetic circulation into your practice of meditation. I thought that in itself was a huge step…

CHAPTER ONE HUNDRED AND FIFTEEN

Subject: Qi Gong Self-Practice - Training 1
Date: Wednesday, April 13, 2022 Minute 59

Dr. K inquired whether what I'd shared 'embodied' Qi Gong?

I responded that there were over a thousand schools of Qi Gong, and every Qi Gong Master really had his unique approach and style.

"So, in many ways, you're getting my unique approach," I said.

Nevertheless, I did feel that what I was sharing was aligned with the central tenants of Qi Gong, at least as it was taught to me.

In truth, my practice of Qi Gong with a fusion of the bioenergy that I had learned that came from the osteopathic approach, and the Qi Gong that I had learned from Master Chou; and I did wonder that I should refer to my approach as 'Bioener-Qi' to exemplify that it is a fusion of the two. At the very least, it was the Bioener-Qi School of Qi Gong.

I noted how it was the Kino had initially questioned me, saying, "You're calling this Qi Gong, but you're not even Chinese?"

And perhaps some would consider this a legitimate point of concern? ("The Jewish guy saying that he's teaching Qi Gong," I said.) Because the last thing I wanted to do was offend anyone's culture and traditions.

In the end I could say that I had undergone extensive Qi Gong training, been certified in this approach by Master Chou, and was trying to be as straight and forthcoming about all this as I could. Perhaps, it could be summed up best this way: This is an energy medicine approach that I've developed based on my 30 years-experience, training in Energy Medicine within multiple disciplines,

cultures and traditions, including Osteopathy, Traditional Chinese Medicine and native healing approaches…

CHAPTER ONE HUNDRED AND SIXTEEN

Subject: Qi Gong Self-Practice - Training 1
Date: Wednesday, April 13, 2022 Minute 102

Bill inquired if I ever considered using this approach to help those with problems of allergies? In response, I told him about an experience early in my training with a child who had difficulties with asthma: Her parents requested my assistance, saying that Dianna's asthma began after she'd had a chest cold. Studying the medical literature I learned that reactive airway disease in children often develops in response to viral infection. I postulated that a viral infection caught Diana's immune system 'off-guard', so that, in response, the immune system was now in a hypervigilant state, 'reacting' and provoking a massive inflammatory reaction to anything remotely resembling a pathogen and resulting in an asthma attack. Indeed, when performing bioenergy with Dianna, I felt an abnormal amount of energy radiating from her chest.

In turn, I developed a four-pronged approach for treatment: 1) Bioenergy to reconcile the body with its previous trauma; 2) Nutrition to strengthen the immune system; 3) Reducing allergen exposure, thereby giving the body time to heal; and, 4) Judicious use of medication to remedy acute attacks. With time Diana got better and her asthma resolved.

Now, I wonder if the same approach can be taken with long COVID? Because really it amounts to the same thing: In COVID-19 there is the trauma of being struck by a foreign virus that the system has never encountered before. In the case of recipients with post-COVID-19 syndrome it would appear that the body is maintaining a hypervigilant state in spite of long-term COVID-19 symptoms being disadvantageous to the body working at its optimal function. At this moment I am working towards investigating the use of bioenergy to treat these recipients, so to reconcile them with the trauma of the COVID-19 infection, rid them of long COVID symptoms and restore them to their prior state of health

And I got back to the earlier discussion with Dr. K about intention, and how this process showed that I had listened to the parents, considered how it was that the child's condition had followed from a viral infection, reviewed the medical literature, postulated the hypothesis that this virus has been a source of trauma to the child system (that it did not know how to come to terms with and reconcile, and as a result it was constantly on guard and hyperalert and reacting to everything that made contact with the upper respiratory system, and, in turn, was doing the system more harm than good), such that there was an 'intention' to affect a communication with the body-mind of the child and say, "I know your system was traumatized in the past by that upper respiratory infection, but you were able to ultimately handle it, and you don't need to be in this hyperalert state, because it's actually doing more harm than good to the person right now. It's time to let go of that."

And it had a good result: The child stopped having asthma attacks. And, indeed, that experience has been the inspiration for me postulating that this approach might help for long Covid which I have plans to perform at UC Davis with the Integrative Medicine Department, Pulmonology Department and Infectious Disease Department there.

That this was the result of the system having been traumatized by this completely new and novel virus that it had never encountered before, and what was needed was for the body-mind to come to terms and reconcile that experience, and perhaps releasing the retained energy of trauma from that experience via this approach would be helpful, and get the system out of being in a hyperalert state that was potentially manifesting in so many other problems.

At the end of this discussion, we concluded the session.

Of note, though, these sessions would lead me to bring the Qi Gong self-practice into the long COVID project…

CHAPTER ONE HUNDRED AND SEVENTEEN

So, Dr. K had her training in virtual Qi Gong.

Now, there was attending to the next request in her email:

"I noticed that we have not worked with someone with an SUD [Substance Use Disorder] and am wondering how this might apply to my patient population?"

Hence, for a second time I was back to the question, Who would serve as test subject?...

CHAPTER ONE HUNDRED AND EIGHTEEN

Now, some years ago, an elderly gentleman showed up at the clinic. His name was Tom. He said he was an author and asked if he could leave a few copies of a book he'd written, titled, "RE-ENTRY Taking Back Your Life", describing difficulties Veterans face getting reacquainted with civilian society and hoping its contents would be helpful to our homeless Veterans?

Then, he inquired whether he could volunteer to help our homeless veterans?

From we'd met, I'd been taken by Tom's gentle, unassuming manner. He struck me as a model of humility – His only interest to be helpful and nothing more.

I was moved and asked if he'd be interested in leading a creative writing group for our homeless veterans, which I'd been trying to get off the ground?

He accepted, and although participants were few, he was not discouraged and became a welcomed fixture in our homeless veteran workgroup.

Over time, I'd get to know him and learn about his life. He had problems of chronic pain and hinted at having had addiction issues, so that it had been in the back of my mind for a while whether bioenergy and Qi Gong might be helpful to him?

It was in this way that Tom came to be the second veteran in our Innovation Accelerator Qi Gong project.

Little did I know at the time, however, that he would bring the project full-circle…

CHAPTER ONE HUNDRED AND NINETEEN

What follows are the notes from the first Qi Gong training session with Tom and Dr. K. I'll try not to make them too 'clinical.' Of note, this and all the other Qi Gong sessions were recorded.

As well as Tom, Dr. K and myself, the other folks present were Addiction Recovery Treatment Services (ARTS) Supervisor, Shelly, and electrostimulation expert, Brian.

For this training session, I am going to keep my voice to a minimum, so to keep the focus on Tom and the others as they navigate the Qi Gong treatment experience.

Again, for those of you interested in learning more about my experience in this area, I refer you to what amounts to my latest reference guide for this healing approach entitled, 'Bioenergy Therapy.'

Getting back to the Qi Gong treatment that follows, I'm going to endeavor to share it in simple, clear and concise language in the hope that that will make these sessions easier to follow.

Of note about this first treatment session with Tom, it turned out that Dr. K had extraordinary, innate energy healing ability, such that she essentially stole the proverbial show in this session (and, in doing so, surprised all of us, including herself). Also notable was the skill and sensitivity that Brian displayed.

And, finally, the reason why Tom's participation in the project would take it full circle is because for the past 25 years Tom had been treated with opioid medications for problems of chronic pain (mostly involving his back and shoulders) and had significant problems of opioid dependence, as well as significant history of substance abuse and self-described "addictive personality."

At the time he was being prescribed hydrocodone twice a day and morphine three times a day. He said he didn't want to be so dependent on these medications, but each time that he attempted to decrease them, he experienced significant symptoms of opioid withdrawal. These withdrawal symptoms included chills; not being able to sleep for more than an hour or two at a time; his arms and legs flailing uncontrollably from the moment he'd lay down to rest; diarrhea; fatigue; loss of appetite because nothing taste good; and extreme pain that was unbearable.

What follows is a rendering of Tom's treatment and response to Qi Gong for his condition.

Subject: Qi Gong in the Treatment of Chronic Pain & Opioid Dependence - Training 1
Date: Wednesday, April 27, 2022 Minute 0
A considerable distance…

The session began with me introducing the different trainees to Tom. Trainees included Qi Gong trainees Dr. K, Shelly and Brian.

Next, I briefly explained Medical Qi Gong to Tom and then offered him the Qi Tangibility Exercise.

Tom scanned above my hand and I asked him what he perceived.

"Heat," he responded.

I asked him where he experienced that heat?

"At the palm," he said.

I then invited Tom to attempt to find a more subtle energy point by scanning over my forearm.

However, Tom was experiencing too much pain in his right shoulder than to be able to continue scanning this way.

"I had a transplanted shoulder," he said indicating the right shoulder.

Of note, Tom hand about a foot above my arm while performing the tangibility exercise, which is a relatively considerable distance and suggested a high acuity for energy perception…

CHAPTER ONE HUNDRED AND TWENTY

Subject: Qi Gong in the Treatment of Chronic Pain & Opioid Dependence - Training 1
Date: Wednesday, April 27, 2022 Minute 4
Drag…

I continued by describing the reason why I performed the tangibility exercise. That this was a rather nebulous practice, and the tangibility exercise gave patients an idea about what I was doing, by being able to locate discrete points of energy over me, before I search their bodies for energy imbalances by scanning for energy disturbances with my hands.

I next proceeded to perform the tangibility exercise with Dr. K.

Dr. K indicated that she could feel discrete points of energy at the palm and the forearm.

"Interesting," she said. "The palm I can also feel like right here with a tingling sensation"

I asked to put out like discrete points?

"Yeah, right here. I can feel it here. And one right there. As though there's a string there, like pulling down."

Next I went to Shelly. she also experienced the energy from the points in the form of tingling.

"A little tingling right there," she said.

I inquired if they felt like discreet points to her as well, and she responded in the affirmative.

Next, I went to Brian.

"I can feel like a drag," Brian said. "Or like you described… A string. More string, I guess. That's a good analogy. And I feel it above your thumb, as well."

I explained again the nature of the tangibility exercise and then the energetics circulation in general. That in its normal state, it flows naturally and uninhibitedly. But when the person experiences trauma, energy collects and gives way to these energy disturbances. And if you help a person read themselves of this retained energy of trauma, it has the potential to facilitate physical healing in general improved well-being…

CHAPTER ONE HUNDRED TWENTY-ONE

Subject: Qi Gong in the Treatment of Chronic Pain & Opioid Dependence - Training 1
Date: Wednesday, April 27, 2022 Minute 8
"I feel it right here…"

Next, I looked for energy imbalances affecting Tom by quickly scanning with my hand over his body.

Right between his shoulders was a significant energy disturbance. As Tom had indicated his main source of pain was in the right shoulder, I was expecting to find more energy radiating from there, and wondered how this unexpected finding would play out for those here for training. Where I was looking for simple energy vectors at the most likely location of injury, as with Kino, it wasn't looking like it was happening.

But as there was nothing to do about it, I invited Dr. K to scan over Tom and see what she found?

Then, to my surprise, Dr. K directed her hands between his shoulders.

"I feel a lot of heat right here," she said. "I feel it right here." It was the same place I'd found it. She wasn't being swayed by Tom's report of symptoms. She was going with her perception and it took her to the same location as me…

CHAPTER ONE HUNDRED TWENTY-TWO

Subject: Qi Gong in the Treatment of Chronic Pain & Opioid Dependence - Training 1
Date: Wednesday, April 27, 2022 Minute 10
Super healer?

I invited Shelly to scan over Tom next.

"I feel it more on this side," Shelly said, indicating Tom's left.

I went back and scanned Tom again, and found that the energy had changed – There was more energy over the left side, and the previous energy disturbance that I had found between the shoulders was no longer there.

I wondered if it had been neutralized by Dr. K and whether Dr. K was just one of these super' energy healers, with an innate gift for this approach, so that all she had to do was connect with an energy disturbance to release the retained energy of trauma there…

CHAPTER ONE HUNDRED TWENTY-THREE

Subject: Qi Gong in the Treatment of Chronic Pain & Opioid Dependence - Training 1
Date: Wednesday, April 27, 2022 Minute 11

I invited Dr. K to go back and see what she felt over Tom now, curious if she'd also perceive something different?

"That's interesting," she said. "It definitely feels different. It feels more to the left. It's definitely cooled down here," she said indicating the location of the previous site of energy disturbance.

Tom talked about his condition and procedures he had undergone.

"I had a shoulder implant on my right side," he began. "And I have a big new German shepherd dog who bounced and polled it out of the socket.

"So they just recently put a new artificial shoulder on the right side. It's not healed yet.

I commented that energy disturbances do not always correlate with patient symptoms.

Nevertheless, Tom indicated that, in general, his left shoulder hurt more than the right…

CHAPTER ONE HUNDRED TWENTY-FOUR

Subject: Qi Gong in the Treatment of Chronic Pain & Opioid Dependence - Training 1
Date: Wednesday, April 27, 2022 Minute 14

I invited Brian to see what he perceived? He localize the energy disturbance to the left shoulder, as well.

"I can definitely feel the heat under the scapula," he said.

I considered neutralizing it myself, but then thought I would test Dr. K to determine if her abilities were as I expected and invited her to attend Tom's energy disturbance?

Immediately, Dr. K demonstrated an ability to perceive directionality with the energy disturbances?

"It feels like it wants to move over," she said, indicating the path of the energy was moving to the left.

I suggested that she simply follow its path.

And doing so (within a few moments) it was as though she was holding the energy like a large ball between both hands.

"What if it leads me out of the room?" she asked, laughing.

I told her it would be okay and offered a long winded explanation about the first time I'd worked with energy disturbances that led me around the room while working with a friend's mother.

Meanwhile, within a few feet of moving out from Tom, Dr. K had followed the energy path to the extent that was needed.

She shook off the feeling from her hands and was quickly back at Tom's side and repeating the process. Again, she went from scanning him to moving the energy outwards, as though carrying some large helium balloon between her hands before letting it go.

"It just feels like I'm pushing it out," she said.

She was: Ridding Tom of the energy disturbance that had been at his left shoulder.

"I'm going back," she said, returning to Tom a third time.

But she found there was nothing left.

"I don't feel it," she announced

Scanning Tom, I found that Dr. K had, indeed, mostly corrected the energy imbalance.

In a matter of minutes, she'd become adept at energy healing…

CHAPTER ONE HUNDRED TWENTY-FIVE

Subject: Qi Gong in the Treatment of Chronic Pain & Opioid Dependence - Training 1
Date: Wednesday, April 27, 2022 Minute 19
'Shift'?...

I invited Brian to see what he perceived. He also indicated that the energy disturbance was no longer present over Tom's shoulder; however, I was observing that Tom was leaning back as Brian was working on him, and Tom also commented about this.

"It was like my body was curving back,"?" Tom said. "And I was wondering about this? It felt like there was someone pulling me back?"

Brian had also observed this.

"And I could see him shift?" Brian said."I could see him."

"Did you feel it?" Tom asked him.

"I could see it," Brian responded." "That you were obviously moving away. Or else you would've touched me. It was interesting."

I admitted that I wondered if Tom was tired and that was the source of his backwards movement?

"Like I was falling asleep," Tom responded, laughing. "No..."

CHAPTER ONE HUNDRED TWENTY-SIX

Subject: Qi Gong in the Treatment of Chronic Pain & Opioid Dependence - Training 1
Date: Wednesday, April 27, 2022 Minute 21

I announced that it was my feeling that we were getting into the realm of the more subtle energy disturbances, which I typically described as being in the ether level, further from the body, like a foot or two away.

His energy disturbances were more subtle and more difficult to detect, but nevertheless, that seem to be what we were dealing with, such that the easier energy disturbances to detect and treat were gone and wondered if this was mostly because of Dr. K's extraordinary ability this way?

"What points are you checking?" Dr. K asked.

I responded that I was just standing over the body, and indeed doing it really quickly so it's not to potentially release any energy disturbances before the trainees could.

I did find one remaining energy disturbance that was closer to Tom's body, and since Shelly seem to be the one who was finding this most challenging, I thought she should have an opportunity, because the other Energy disturbances were just becoming more and more difficult.

But when Shelly didn't seem to perceive much, I invited Dr. K next to evaluate.

"Again, I'm feeling pushed," Dr. K said.

She was running out of space.

"I don't know where to go?" she said.

This time I told her succinctly what to do when she ran out of space: She didn't have to worry, saying that if she ran out of space, so that her hand was left to be against the wall, then to just keep on perceiving the energy with her hand there, and let the energy direct her within the limitations of the room.

"If you can't follow it anymore, just stay with it," I said. "A lot of times it would just feel like it is solidly in your hand and that's as far as it wants to go and as much as it wants to do."

"I feel like it is solidly in my hand," she responded.

Then the energy directed her to move.

"I want to do it this way," she indicated as the energy seem to be turning her in a clockwise fashion.

She laughed.

"I will say, internally, I'm like, 'I wonder what I am going to do with this if it doesn't leave me?'"

I assured her that she could always just wash her hands if she didn't want to let the energy just disappeared on its own. Indeed, that's how I was trained when it came to working with these energy disturbances at first.

"Yeah, I'm starting to feel like anxious," she said. "I think that what I worry about with Energy Work is taking it with me – I might absorb it."

Although acknowledging her fears, I stated that in the thirty years that I'd been doing this work, I'd never had a bad experience that way. Indeed (quite on the contrary) I'd only had good ones.

"If it ever did get into my system," I began, "it only did good things, in terms of activating a similar trauma and retained energy of trauma that me and the recipient shared, so as to move that retained energy of trauma in me from a chronic dormant state to one that was activated and a cute and amenable to healing - So that the retained energy of trauma that I shared with the recipient was now amenable to healing, and the healing could occur inside of me, and I could go back and help the recipient now. Such that I look forward to these experiences.

And though there had been Qi Gong masters with whom I'd trained who had warned that the energy could infect you in a harmful way, experience had taught me over and over again that this form of healing only encompasses healing, not only for the recipient, but also for the practitioner.

I described the fiber optic cable between computers syncing and that working the same way when we connect with the energetics circulation of a patient. The systems are looking for damage programs to correct, and not only in the recipient, but also in the

practitioner – so to make that practitioner a better channel for healing.

"Because that was in the recipient's best interest," I declared. "To make you an even better healer…"

CHAPTER ONE HUNDRED TWENTY-SEVEN

Subject: Qi Gong in the Treatment of Chronic Pain & Opioid Dependence - Training 1
Date: Wednesday, April 27, 2022 Minute 30
'Wondering…"

"It's interesting," Brian commented of Dr. K. "Because as she moved further and further away, it's like it got larger and heavier. And then it dissipated. I could see it in your posture and your movement."

"I felt compelled to use breath work," Dr. K stated. "It was like something was saying to do whatever was viable."

Nodding, I thought she'd done exactly the right thing. Indeed, breath work was something that I regarded myself as deficient – though I could say that between the first Qi Gong recording (when my lungs were so tight that I could hardly mumble a sentence without the need to take another breath) and now, I was improving with every Qi Gong session.

Meanwhile, for all her innate ability, where Dr. K had voiced concerns about Tom's energy not 'leaving' her, I wondered aloud if perhaps Dr. K wanted to take a step back from doing anymore?

But she indicated that she wanted to continue.

"I think it's important to talk about it," she said. "Because I got anxious."

She laughed.

"And I wouldn't say that I'm necessarily worried," she added. "But I'm wondering?…"

CHAPTER ONE HUNDRED TWENTY-EIGHT

Subject: Qi Gong in the Treatment of Chronic Pain & Opioid Dependence - Training 1
Date: Wednesday, April 27, 2022 Minute 35
"Like I'm holding helium…"

Scanning Tom, it felt as though his crown chakra had opened, and I invited the others to experience it, starting with Shelly, who seemed to me required more training than the others.

"I'm getting like tingling feelings, at the top of my head," Shelly said.

Dr. K looked at me.

"Do you ever go in sync?" Dr. K asked, insightfully. "Like if somebody's crown chakra opens, does it feel like yours opens as well?"

I think this work opens my crown chakra, in general. It's probably the reason I experience a sense of awe and reverence every time I connect with another's energetic circulation.

Meanwhile, I asked Shelly if the experience was uncomfortable?

"No, it's not in a bad way," she said. "It just feels kind of cool and fluid. Almost like there were a jagged quality and not just one that feels kind of soft."

I invited Dr. K to see what she experienced?

"It does feel very light," she commented. "It's almost like helium. Like I'm holding helium."

Tom indicated that he was feeling stiff and wanted to stand and stretch for a moment.

When he sat again, I went back and evaluated him, and found that I was unable to locate any energy over his head, as though anything I'd previously perceived over his crown chakra was gone.

"Did I do something?" Dr. K asked.

Yes, it seemed she had.

She apologized.

But there was nothing to apologize for. She was simply an energy healing machine…

CHAPTER ONE HUNDRED TWENTY-NINE

Subject: Qi Gong in the Treatment of Chronic Pain & Opioid Dependence - Training 1
Date: Wednesday, April 27, 2022 Minute 38

"I still feel the warmth here," Brian said, indicating Tom's left shoulder. "But I don't feel the push. It feels smooth but warm. Less jagged."

"I feel like asking if Qi Gong follows certain channels or meridians or chakras?" Dr. K asked. "Because you seem to teach more intuitively. Like just go to where it is, and get out of your head as to where it's at. Is that correct?"

Yes, I would say that was correct. I felt that something that made Qi Gong different from tai chi and acupuncture and other forms of traditional Chinese medicine was the free-flowing nature of Qi Gong. This was a practice that really got in touch with the energy at basest level – One that was not prescribed. We were dealing with the body's response to individual trauma, and therefore treating it at a level that was completely unique to the individual – For which there was no standard approach. No standard set of movements. No standard set of acupuncture points to use. No standard set of meridians to incorporate. Just working with the patient's energy disturbance at a completely individual and unique way.

It was my feeling that Qi Gong was the father of all of the other TCM practices, like tai chi and acupuncture, etc., which came out of 'bystander' effects – meaning, that as individual healing was occurring in the practice of Qi Gong, the Qi Gong masters were finding that certain postures and points and meridians and channels helped with just about everything, and thereby could be used to offer

broad-based exercises, postures, breathing practices, etc. that could help the general public, especially those who we're not as adept at perceiving the energetic circulation or as well-versed and positioned in society to receive training in Qi Gong.

"These other approaches (Tai Chi, etc.) not do as much for linking the person to the universal Chi, so to really focus on their unique and individual energy disturbances," I said, "but they would do something to serve as an exercise for moving the energy around, enhancing with energy reserves within the body, especially for when the system became depleted, and facilitate healing..."

CHAPTER ONE HUNDRED THIRTY

Subject: Qi Gong in the Treatment of Chronic Pain & Opioid Dependence - Training 1
Date: Wednesday, April 27, 2022 Minute 45

As Brian energetically attended Tom, I noted a very interesting phenomenon of Tom leaning backwards, as though being pulled in the direction of Brian's hands.

"I felt like I was pulling him a little bit again,", Brian said and shrugged. "Did you feel like I was pulling you?"

I asked Brian if he would identify where he was perceiving the energy blockage on Tom, and as soon as Brian did that, Tom went right back into that lean.

And Tom didn't demonstrate the least discomfort, despite the position looking precarious; i.e., an elderly man leaning half way back?

And as soon as Brian moved his hands away, Tom went right back to his original erect sitting position.

"It's right between the scapula," Brian stated. "Maybe a little bit lateral."

Scanning over Tom, I identified an energy disturbance at that location; however, with me, Tom did not exhibit any of the leaning behavior that he had with Brian, and I postulated that Brian was reaching Tom at a unique energy frequency, so to trigger this response?...

CHAPTER ONE HUNDRED THIRTY-ONE

Subject: Qi Gong in the Treatment of Chronic Pain & Opioid Dependence - Training 1
Date: Wednesday, April 27 2022 Minute 49

Tom commented that he thought the source of what we were seeing with his back was related to opioid medications and previous behavior.

"I used to work out with weights at an older age," he professed. "I was also taking opiates and then lifting weights, which was a dumb thing to do. Because I think what happened was that I just wore out my major joints – knees, shoulders, the back.

I stood with my head down: I thought this is one of the worst problems when it came to treating a patient with opiates; that being, when patients are on that medication, they don't know what their limits are, so that by treating their pain, the doctor can wind up making these patients' condition even worse!

"That's against the very heart of Hippocrates oath," I said. "'Primum non nocere – First do no harm.' Those providers essentially did Tom harm…"

CHAPTER ONE HUNDRED THIRTY-TWO

Subject: Qi Gong in the Treatment of Chronic Pain & Opioid Dependence - Training 1
Date: Wednesday, April 27, 2022 Minute 55
Heart chakra…

Feeling energy emanating from chakras midline across Tom's body, I invited Shelly to feel for energy chakras midline over Tom; however, it seemed too subtle for her.

Brian was next and he felt maybe a little, but again the subtle nature was really beyond his ability to work with.

Then I invited Dr. K to try, if she felt up to it?

"I can give it a try," she said.

She was standing a considerable distance from Tom when she began, maybe some two or three feet away. Nevertheless, shortly upon scanning Tom, she commented, "I feel like I'm being pushed. It feels like I need to be out here," indicating even further from him.

Her acuity for energy perception was simply extraordinary – higher than any beginner I'd ever worked with before. Perceiving energy imbalances at this distance just wasn't the norm for someone who'd just been introduced to this approach. Most beginners typically only perceive energy disturbances that are 'vector'-like and radiating intensely at a short distance from the patient's body. In that way, Shelly's and Brian's experience was much more in keeping with that.

Nevertheless, I continued, commenting that I had been feeling something from the heart chakra originally, and then at the third eye.

"This feels like something," she said. "Like my left hand feels heavy. I don't know what to say more than that. Not feeling like it's his energy, but feeling like I could topple on this," she indicated her left side.

"Just because you can sense it, does it mean that the energy is trying to do something with you?" she asked. "Because sometimes that perception is just like that push or a pull, or like it's not guiding you anywhere."

I responded that, in general, I didn't try to interpret the meaning of the energy path or corresponding sensations.

"Then just your presence is therapeutic?" she asked. "Just your feeling the jagged heat? If it's not giving you the directionality?"

Yes, it was about making an energetic connection, so to gain your help in facilitating the release of retained energy of trauma or figuring through where trauma had left it dysfunctional and how it could regain or optimize that function again.

Brian (who was also quite innately gifted in this area) offered additional insights.

"When you were against the wall," Brian said, "it physically turned you towards the wall - Which was amazing! I watched it. You remember you said, 'It wants to take me this way.' It did."

Meanwhile, Shelly had been scanning Tom and indicated that she perceived a "presence around the heart."

"Maybe it's my pacemaker," Tom responded. "I'm 100% pacemaker dependent - Which I'm going to a checkup for at 3:30 today."

Though I didn't think it was electrical activity from the pacemaker that we were perceiving, I would later have significant conversations with Tom about how it was that a heart condition inspired his spiritual path…

CHAPTER ONE HUNDRED THIRTY-THREE

Subject: Qi Gong in the Treatment of Chronic Pain & Opioid Dependence - Training 1
Date: Wednesday, April 27, 2022 Minute 1:03
Trusting one's feelings…

It seemed an energy shell was evolving around Tom that was pushing me further and further back (Not unlike what Dr. K had experienced), so to suggest that we had come to the end of the Qi Gong treatment.

I invited the others to potentially experience this energy shell. Dr. K was the first to volunteer.

"Interesting," she commented. "Yeah, there are not focal points."

Dr. K had commented that she was feeling tired, but didn't feel that acting on it was "patient centric."

I disagreed, saying that by listening to your own body, it might be that it would ultimately lead her to a place of becoming a better healer and, thus, better be able to help patients.

I talked about my own journey about experiencing the funny buzz with some patients and that taking me to Qi Gong, and how learning to self-practice led me to overcome that 'funny buzz'; and discovered that the 'funny buzz' was alerting me to a place of retained energy of trauma in my system that was similar to the patient and getting in the way of me being an effective healer and being able to help that patient; such that if I addressed that retained energy of trauma via self-maintenance Qi Gong, I would rid myself of that 'turbid Qi', so to be able to get back to the patient and help that patient now.

Ergo, by listening to my body when it was telling me that I needed to do something for myself, it ultimately led me to be able to help my patients better.

So, if she felt like she needed some rest, then I would trust her judgment and trust her feelings, and perhaps that would help her integrate the experiences from this session, so to become better at this energy work…

CHAPTER ONE HUNDRED THIRTY-FOUR

Subject: Qi Gong in the Treatment of Chronic Pain & Opioid Dependence - Training 1
Date: Wednesday, April 27, 2022 Minute 108

Tom described having experiencing beneficial effects from the session, declaring, "Now I know why dogs like to be petted. I feel more energy. Like I've been petted. I feel lighter right now. Peaceful. I feel good. Like I'm ready to hit the road.

He inquired whether his pacemaker might be a source of detected energy in the session? My feeling was it wasn't, asserting that Qi Gong worked with the endogenously energies of the body, and not those of an electronic device.

"They aren't what we evolved to work when it comes to this work," I said of the pacemaker. "It really seems like we're meant to help each other with each other's energies."

"Well, I thank you for your energies," Tom said graciously, as the session concluded…

CHAPTER ONE HUNDRED THIRTY-FIVE

Subject: Qi Gong in the Treatment of Chronic Pain & Opioid Dependence - Post-session interview
Date: Friday, April 29, 2022
"…Felt better. Less pain…"

I reached Tom a couple days after the Qi Gong session.

"It's been a long haul for me," he began. "It started out with scoliosis of my spine and various treatments for that. And then later when the doctor started prescribing opiates, then I decided, 'Well, I'll take the opiates before I go work out with weights', which was about the dumbest thing I could do. And I did that into my 70s. And eventually I just wore out all the joints. It's just like an old car, you know. So that's what happened, and here I am…"

"I had to go after that for a pacemaker check at Kaiser," he continued. "That's why I had to leave early. And when I was driving over there, I all of a sudden realized that I felt much less pain, and the feeling of feeling better was not like feeling better when I take the opiates. It was a different kind of feeling. It was a more normal, smooth feeling. Not like a 'high', and I really felt like I felt better. Less pain."

"It's just felt like a more natural less pain than opiates," he added. "When opiates get rid of the pain, it gives you a little bit of a high. And I didn't feel that at all. It was just like a smooth feeling. And it went on until this morning. And I still feel it somewhat now."

"My focus is better," he continued. "I noticed that. And I feel mentally more like myself. It's subtle. But it's definitely better. There still might be some now. When I went for a walk with my friends, we did our usual two laps. And I'm feeling pretty good."

He inquired about the trainees.

"Those people who practiced on me have done this before, right?" he asked. "The ones who were there yesterday?"

When I responded that it was their first time, he was surprised.

"Really?!" he said. "Because they were impressive. I thought they were very good. I thought they had done it before…"

He described the sense of 'magnetism' that he experienced with Brian.

"The guy - the one who deals with the device you were talking about [Sequential Stimulator]. With him, the movement was strange. It was almost like magnetic. I just felt like a subtle magnetism sort of pulling me back. My spinal cord and bones are all smooth and don't hold. They are very off. So that could've been it. But I don't know why? It didn't happen with any of the other people. And then he did it again for a second time. So, I don't know. It's odd. It almost felt like there was a slight magnetism pulling my body…"

CHAPTER ONE HUNDRED THIRTY-SIX

Subject: Qi Gong in the Treatment of Chronic Pain & Opioid Dependence - Training 2
Date: Wednesday, May 25, 2022 Minute 0

Tom shared that the last Qi Gong session had helped him significantly with pain.

"The shoulder is bone-on-bone," he said, indicating the left shoulder. "This is an implant," he said indicating the right. "So, during the implant, I had to use this [left] shoulder, and now it's pooping out."

Of the previous Qi Gong session, Tom said this:

"I can't explain whether it was a coincidence the effect that Qi Gong had on me," he said. "It was not only physical, although regarding the physical part, my pain is way, way down, It was sort of a feeling of 'myself.' In I felt mentally and physically like I was a couple of decades younger. And my perception seemed cleaner and clearer. It was terrific. I mean, I'm very grateful for it, and it's good to know that it's possible to live without pain again."

Tom did admit that his pain was coming back.

"Mostly in my back and shoulders," he said…

CHAPTER ONE HUNDRED THIRTY-SEVEN

Subject: Qi Gong in the Treatment of Chronic Pain & Opioid Dependence - Training 2
Date: Wednesday, May 25, 2022 Minute 3

Then, Tom addressed me, saying, "You lived with pain for a while, didn't you?"

I responded by telling him the story about my problems of trauma and chronic pain and then finding Qi Gong.

Back then, I was a medical student, I was a graduate student, I was working in science.

I had no thought of doing anything outside the conventional realm.

But conventional medicine wasn't helping.

And when it comes to bioenergy, it was like a lightbulb came on in my head.

"Wow, can I learn more about this?

And Dr. Rind agreed to teach me.

At the same time, I was really leery about doing this within the conventional realm. Afterall, this was a healing approach that involve perceiving what as yet could not be measured, such that there wasn't a way of quantifying bioenergy.

"Kind of far out," he interjected. "Though I'm not a scientist, so I don't know. but I also believe a lot of other things, too. I'm beginning to wonder if the universe has a consciousness?..."

CHAPTER ONE HUNDRED THIRTY-EIGHT

Subject: Qi Gong in the Treatment of Chronic Pain & Opioid Dependence - Training 2
Date: Wednesday, May 25, 2022 Minute 7

Meanwhile, of continued interest to me was that, in the last Qi Gong session, Tom had demonstrated a certain leaning back that hadn't responded to attempts to energetically neutralize the source and fully correct.

Tom described a link between his shoulders and knees, such that when he couldn't use his knees without supporting himself with his shoulders (when either sitting down or attempting to stand up) and this aggravated the pain in his shoulders.

Of Qi Gong in general, Tom commented, "You got to feel it to believe it."

"I always knew that you wouldn't do something that wasn't good for your patients," he said of the Qi Gong expert, "but I did feel it was kind of 'far out', and scientifically… Well, I don't know."

Just prior to the start of today's Qi Gong session, Tom shared that his wife had PTSD and that it had gotten worse.

"She has obsessive compulsive disorder, as well," he said. "When she says yes, she means no. When I tell her to turn left, she turns right. And it's getting worse. And it's not easy for me, because it takes up a lot of my time.

"But I think, 'When you get married, you take an oath, for better or worse, to go through thick and thin, and all that, and I think, maybe that's meant to be my purpose here?... Is to be able to support her through this.

"I have a stepson, but I think if I wasn't here, he'd probably put her in a nursing home. She's physically fine and in good health. It's just changed my life because my day is filled up with doing dishes and picking up, and every five minutes she's asking, 'Tom, can you help me with this thing? Can you help me with that?' And that's my life sort of. I think I'd like to get away for a few days and learn more about these respite things through the VA…"

CHAPTER ONE HUNDRED THIRTY-NINE

Subject: Qi Gong in the Treatment of Chronic Pain & Opioid Dependence - Training 2
Date: Wednesday, May 25, 2022 Minute 12

The Qi Gong session began with a demonstration of Qi via the Qi Tangibility Exercise. As well as Tom feeling the energy at my palm, Tom demonstrated significant directionality perception, indicating of the energy, "It feels like it's guiding my hand up."

Tom inquired of the Qi Gong expert whether performing Qi Gong "depletes your energy?" or if it took any energy from me to do this kind of work? I responded that it was just the opposite; that I found performing Qi Gong was extraordinarily rejuvenating, and that the moment I tap into another's energetic circulation, I enter a place of awe and reverence for the person that I find rejuvenating and a joy...

Prior to initiating the Qi Gong treatment, I made sure the Tom was comfortable, and he asked that the head of the examination table be inclined, and I did so.

Starting at his left side, it quickly moved me to his right, as I follow the energy at high speed. This would be very different from later in the session, when the energy would move exceedingly slowly.

Shortly after we began the Qi Gong treatment, Tom said that he had the experience of spinning.

"It's not so much vertigo, as feeling like I'm swimming around," he said.

I was reminded me of the energy whirlpool that Bill found while working with Kino a couple of weeks ago (for which I, in turn, enjoyed the experience of entering and then neutralizing).

"It's like I'm connected to your hand," Tom continued, "and I feel the movement of you through the air… As you moved, I felt something... Energy... With your movement. And even though you're not touching me, I feel this molding. In my chest. In my head. If you're going down, I sort of feel that. It's like I was maybe a big pole in the barber shop – with stripes the way it goes around it, and I'm like the pole you're feeling."

"I feel like you are almost petting an invisible dog," he continued, "And I'm the dog getting petted. Like we're connected. While you're not touching me, it feels like you're almost petting or massaging the energy in some way, and it makes me feel like the petted dog."

"It feels good," he added. "It feels comforting and reassuring."

At the time the energy was moving exceedingly slowly. I alerted Tom, and indicated that in spite of the potential monotony I was going to continue to follow the energy at the speed that it directed.

"I still feel like the invisible dog being petted," Tom asserted. "I feel like there's something out there. Or something emanating from me that is not visible, but that I can feel it, and perhaps you can feel it? And that's like being petted…"

CHAPTER ONE HUNDRED FORTY

Subject: Qi Gong in the Treatment of Chronic Pain & Opioid Dependence - Training 2
Date: Wednesday, May 25, 2022 Minute 24

When I inquired about the "emanating" feeling and whether he thought it was energy, he responded, "Yes, I do, but it's a slow flow. It's mainly coming out from my heart, or the middle of my body."

Of note, at the same time that I was experiencing that excruciatingly slow progress in following the path of the energy from Tom, he'd made this comment of a 'slow flow'...

I asked if Tom was familiar with the chakras, because it sounded like a chakra experience?

He said that he was familiar, and it felt like it was a chakra experience to him, too, and it was a good feeling.

"It feels good," he said of the energy healing experience. "It feels almost like a massage maybe?"

Of note, 'external' Qi Gong was also referred to as 'Qi Gong massage.'

"Have you ever seen someone pulling taffy?" he asked. "It's kind of like that in a way."

"What I feel is that the energy is following your hand," he continued. "It's not just the energy being there.

"And it's happening at the heart chakra," he added. "It's weird..."

CHAPTER ONE HUNDRED FORTY-ONE

Subject: Qi Gong in the Treatment of Chronic Pain & Opioid Dependence - Training 2
Date: Wednesday, May 25, 2022 Minute 28

I had been squatting for a long time. When I went back to evaluate, the energy move from Tom's heart chakra moved outwards and then to the right of the room.

Coming back to Tom again, the energy move from tom's heart chakra and then arced downwards into the ground

"I feel the energy less centered and going lower," Tom said. "The lower portion of my body. At below my navel here.

It sounded like he was referring to the Lower Dantien. I explained that in Traditional Chinese Medicine (TCM), the Lower Dantien was located just below the navel. It was perhaps the most important of the energy centers in TCM, associated with the first place that we breathe, that being through the umbilicus via the umbilical cord when life begins in the womb.

"I definitely feel it there," he asserted.

Of note, in TCM, the heart chakra is referred to as the Middle Dantien. In this way, the movement of his energy had gone from Middle Dantien to Lower Dantien.

As this was occurring, it was my experience that Tom's energy was arcing to the ground, which I interpreted as the retained energy of trauma (so-called 'turbid Qi') moving to the soil where it could feed mother earth, and explained the 'Waterfall effect', which was explained in detail when I similar phenomenon occurred with Kino last week.

Tom commented that he could imagine that it was a lot of retained energy of trauma when it came to Kino, "considering what he went through," he said.

I would learn that Tom had been through a lot of trauma, too…

CHAPTER ONE HUNDRED FORTY-TWO

Subject: Qi Gong in the Treatment of Chronic Pain & Opioid Dependence - Training 2
Date: Wednesday, May 25, 2022 Minute 35

Tom commented on his impression of Kino based on seeing him today.

"He really looks healthy and happy," he said. "Like he's feeling happier than the way he did before the accident."

I confided how it was that at the time of Kino's accident in 2018, I'd been very busy traveling back-and-forth between Sacramento and Redding, attending to matters related to the opioid crisis; however, every moment that I wasn't on the road, I spent visiting with Kino in the hospital during the weeks that he was in a coma and then on the ward recuperating.

It was a deeply touching personal experience, I said. Memories that I would never forget.

"He went through a lot," Tom repeated...

Tom said he was becoming aware of a feeling in his head.

"It feels like it's pulsating," he said. "In the forehead and in the temples.

"I also feel the pulse of my heart more. I'm usually not aware of the pulse of my heart - But I feel it.

"I feel my heart beating, but I also feel like the veins and the capillaries are getting fuller, filling up the empty spaces

"I sort of feel like the heart chakra is opening a bit."

I thought it might be that his third eye chakra becoming activated, and (at the risk of being accused leading the participant) I inquired if he felt like what was going on?

"I don't know," he responded. "It's there where the third eye is, in the middle of the forehead."

I wanted to explore about what might be going on where these chakra activations were concerned: I thought it was likely related to feelings revolving around his concern for his wife, but first I wanted to inquire about feeling related to his pacemaker, since he'd mentioned about his pacemaker during the active Qi Gong session, and only talked about his wife before the active Qi Gong session.

So I asked if the cardiac pacemaker took up a lot of his awareness?

"None," he responded, definitively. "It is such a blessing. I remember when I first got it, which was a long time ago – I was 42 or 43 years old - and since then I've been totally unaware of any problems with it. They always want me to monitor it at home and attach me to all these electronic devices, and I say, 'No, if it's working, fine. If it doesn't, I die. Why do I want to preoccupy myself about it? You worry about it!'"

He laughed.

"The pacemaker, it's incredible," he said. "If you ever have to get one, be thankful. It's not a bad thing."

Tom commented about how it is that someone could monitor the pacemaker without touching you, and I went into an exploration of how it is that Qi Gong might offer a similar means of connecting with someone and looking for energy imbalances 'without touching you', but connecting via the energetics circulation and syncing like a couple of computers to attend damaged programs (This theory has been previously discussed in the seventh Qi Gong Training session.)

"It's just like the way they read the pacemaker – and didn't touch me," Tom commented. "There's some connection there - It's just an invisible connection."

Yes, just like assessing and evaluating the status of the pacemaker through the phone, the energetic circulation represented that invisible connection when I worked on people via Qi Gong.

That was one theory as to how it worked…

CHAPTER ONE HUNDRED FORTY-THREE

Subject: Qi Gong in the Treatment of Chronic Pain & Opioid Dependence - Training 2
Date: Wednesday, May 25, 2022 Minute 51

Tom described experiencing a new energy sensation involving his heart chakra, so to describe a feeling like energy was coming from him and going straight ahead.

"It feels like it's sending and receiving," he said. "It's almost like breathing underwater. Of something that expels the water and then fills it back in. And it flows back and forth. Like underwater photography, where you're on the seafloor in the seaweed, and the current goes back-and-forth like this. The natural current."

The energy was taking me back to Tom.

"I feel heat," he said.

Indeed, I was feeling energy emanating from my hands.

Then, he commented that he'd experienced the energy "became very strong for a moment."

"It shook my nerves," he said and chuckled good-naturedly. "I felt like the energy was so strong, like it was coming too fast."

I attempted to reassure him that I had not purposely directed any energy towards him; I was just following the energy, whether it was taking me away from him, or whether it was taking me towards him. I was simply following it at all times in a passive way. There was never any intention or thought like, Let's hit Tom with a lot of energy at once.

"'Let's zap him'," Tom added, laughing and joking.

At the same time, it felt like the energy was taking me back to Tom, so that my hands were relatively close to him and felt charged

with energy and asked if he had any perception of feeling energy coming from me?

"Yes," he responded. "I feel heat. Like you're holding an energy wand…"

CHAPTER ONE HUNDRED FORTY-FOUR

Subject: Qi Gong in the Treatment of Chronic Pain & Opioid Dependence - Training 2
Date: Wednesday, May 25, 2022 Minute 57

Tom indicated that he wanted a break to get up, as he'd been sitting for a while.

When he stood up, he commented about how it was that he was able to do it without a cane.

"Usually I need a cane to do that," he said.

He walked about the room. (As for me, the energy was holding me in a kneeling position.)

Tom stretched so as to nearly touch his toes, and then straightened again.

Returning to the examination table, he sat unassisted without the use of the cane and without supporting himself with his upper body.

"I sat down with my legs only," he commented. "I didn't have to brace myself, which I usually do, both getting up and sitting down."

He commented how it was that bracing himself to sit using his upper body led to pain and difficulties in his shoulders (which he'd also commented on prior to the active Qi Gong session).

He laughed.

"I don't know," he continued. "I don't want to get my hopes too high, but I feel pretty good. I feel hopeful. I get the feeling that this has been very helpful. If it's anything like last time, I have some good times ahead…"

CHAPTER ONE HUNDRED FORTY-FIVE

Subject: Qi Gong in the Treatment of Chronic Pain & Opioid Dependence - Training 2
Date: Wednesday, May 25, 2022 Minute 59

"I feel it was a very good session and I look forward to the time ahead."

Indeed, the following day, he would report that he'd continued to walk unassisted and without the assistance of a cane, and feeling significantly better.

I offered to teach Tom the Qi Gong self-practice technique, but he indicated that he wanted to get going, and commented some more about his concerns regarding his wife.

"I always worry about my wife. She's so dependent," he said. "It's pretty much nonstop. I feel like when I'm not doing anything…"

He broke off and said that he better get back to her.

"She had an accident last night," he said. "A fall. At the front door…."

He inquired how long we have been doing this? When the timer indicated that it turned out the session had lasted about an hour, both of us were surprised, and neither felt it had been that long."

Again, the day after this Qi Gong session, Tom declared that he did not need to use his cane for walking and his pain was significantly diminished….

CHAPTER ONE HUNDRED FORTY-SIX

Subject: Qi Gong in the Treatment of Chronic Pain & Opioid Dependence - Training 2
Date: Wednesday, June 1, 2022 Minute 0

In this Qi Gong training session of the Innovation Accelerator project, the 85-year old Veteran with chronic pain was taken through a Qi Gong self-practice session.

The week before this session, the Veteran had said the following of his Qi Gong experiences:

"The first time [on April 27, 2022] it made a big difference with my pain level," he said. "This last time [May 25, 2022], not so much, although it was down. And it's been down. But what it has done, is it sort of done something with my mind or my spirit or something, where I want to do things again that I couldn't do before - I wouldn't do before. And I have more energy to want to do creative things then I've had in a couple of years, and that feels really good."

Now, before beginning this session, the Veteran again related that he had received significant relief of pain through Qi Gong, then indicated he was looking for a Qi Gong to help with problems in his major joints.

"After my first session, I had quite a bit of relief for a week or so," he stated. "The pain is now back in my shoulders, my knees and my back. And that would be the major thing for me.

"Second, is energy. I feel that something happened to me with the Qi Gong sessions, so that I got my ability back as a writer. I had writer's block for two years. I don't know. I quit doing it. And since doing this, I've kind of reverted back to my mental state from a few years ago, so that I have more drive to be creative; and I've kind of

broken that barrier; and I'm very grateful for. I didn't think such a thing was really possible, and it was just my age. So, I think it's great."

Just before the Qi Gong expert was about to initiate a Qi Gong healing session, the Veteran commented that he hadn't been practicing Qi Gong at home; in response, the Qi Gong expert commented that the Veteran had not been trained in Qi Gong self-practice.

"No, and I want to," the Veteran responded. "Because I think it will make these sessions more meaningful."

The Qi Gong expert offered to take the Veteran through a Qi Gong self-practice, and veteran responded in the affirmative.

"I would love it," he said…

CHAPTER ONE HUNDRED FORTY-SEVEN

Subject: Qi Gong in the Treatment of Chronic Pain & Opioid Dependence - Training 3
Date: Wednesday, June 1, 2022 Minute 3

The Qi Gong expert took a chair next to the Veteran and initiated the Qi Gong self-practice, starting with the ball of energy exercise:

1. Centering yourself, seated comfortably and breathing through your nostrils, place your hands (palms facing each other) about 6 inches apart.
2. Imagine that you are holding an energy ball between them and see if you don't perceive some energy at your palms.
3. The energy can take the form of heat or static electricity or tingling at your fingertips or coolness or throbbing or puffs of air or a breeze or feeling of 'magnetic' attraction or repulsion.
4. Feel around the contours of the ball by rolling it around in your hands, back-and-forth.
5. Do this for several minutes.

Next, the Qi Gong expert guided the Veteran through the 'Crown Chakra' element:

5. Start with the 'Ball of Energy' exercise.
6. Once you have a good feeling for the 'ball of energy', move your hands apart and to your sides, still perceiving the energy cupped within your palms.

7. Next, lift your hands slowly above your head. As your hands ascend, feel the energy transferring from them to your head, until you feel energy radiating from the top of your skull. This area of the skull is referred to as the 'seventh chakra' or 'crown chakra.' This chakra connects us with the universe and kindles our desire for spirituality and achieving universal ideals like unconditional love. When this chakra is activated, it promotes a feeling of reverence. This should be a pleasurable experience, leaving you feeling centered, tethered by an energetic string between the crown chakra and the universe, in tune with the energy of the Universe. Of note, it happens that imbalances in the crown chakra occur in response to traumatic experiences, which cause us to wall ourselves off; activating this chakra helps us release the retained energy of trauma and embrace love and comfort.

8. With the crown chakra now activated, bring your hands back to your sides and sit experiencing the energy radiating upwards from your hands and crown chakra for several minutes until the feeling dissipates. If Qi is perceived at the palms as having a directional quality, then follow it with your hands.

The Veteran indicated that he had difficulties lifting his hands because of problems in his shoulders, and the Qi Gong expert instructed him to just lift them to the extent that was comfortable for the Veteran and no further.

The Veteran then requested that the practice be re-started from the beginning, and the Qi Gong expert complied.

The Veteran described "feeling a triangle between my hands and a heart chakra and I can still feel a connection at the top of my head."

Then, as the self-practice continued, the Veteran described feeling "clean."

"I feel the energy at my head going up," he said and laughed. "I feel like I can stay with this energy for a long time."

"I feel like everything and nothing," the Veteran continued. "Everything in the energy is OK, and I don't know what it is - But it is! You're not in control. You're part of the whole."

The Veteran's comment rekindled previous thoughts shared by the Qi Gong expert in which he attempted to describe his experience:

"I believe when I lose myself in others, I get more connected to the whole…"

CHAPTER ONE HUNDRED FORTY-EIGHT

Subject: Qi Gong in the Treatment of Chronic Pain & Opioid Dependence - Training 3
Date: Wednesday, June 1, 2022 Minute 12

"I still feel the energy flowing upwards," the Veteran commented. "I guess it will take a long time for me to empty," alluding to the Qi Gong expert's comments about this practice working to release the retained energy of trauma to the Universal Qi, and laughed.

He described the feeling of energy in his hands.

"I feel it in the palms – in my hands," he said. "It's like I'm holding something, but it isn't heavy."

"I feel particularly like there's something in the palms of my hands," he added, "and it's sort of revolving and moving about."

The Qi Gong expert described his experience of feeling pillars of energy in his hands as well as at the top of his head that seemed to be bringing the energy upwards.

The Veteran, however, described a more gaseous experience.

"I feel like there are chimneys, actually," he said. "Going from my palms and my head and the energy going up from there…"

CHAPTER ONE HUNDRED FORTY-NINE

Subject: Qi Gong in the Treatment of Chronic Pain & Opioid Dependence - Training 3
Date: Wednesday, June 1, 2022 Minute 20

The Veteran also described sensations at the bottom of his feet.

"Sort of the tingling there," he said.

The Qi Gong expert offered to expand the self-practice to bring in "mother earth" energy; however, the veteran declined.

"I think this is enough," he said. "I don't want to go too far. I'd like to save it for another time."

"This has been a satisfying experience," he continued. "More than I had before. I didn't feel the energy in my palms then. I tried it a few times at home, and I didn't feel it as strong or as much as I do now. This has been helpful. I'd like to practice this at my home."

The Qi Gong expert told the Veteran that he leading self-practice sessions virtually on Mondays from his office and invited the Veteran to attend these sessions.

Veteran indicated that he would like to do this with the Qi Gong expert in-person.

"I know virtually is the thing now, but I'm old-fashioned," he said...

Veteran indicated that he received significant benefit from the self-practice session.

"I feel refreshed and connected," he said. "I felt it. I felt a release. I felt connected. I definitely felt connected."

Although the Veteran indicated that he was still actively having an energetic experience, he voiced a desire to end the self-practice

session, and asked that the recording be stopped, so that he could share some personal thoughts with the Qi Gong expert.

This was done, so that the self-practice session concluded…

CHAPTER ONE HUNDRED FIFTY

Subject: Qi Gong in the Treatment of Chronic Pain & Opioid Dependence - Training 4
Date: Wednesday, August 17, 2022 Minute 16

In initiating the Qi Gong training session, I checked in with Tom. Tom described a significant loss: He had been informed recently that a dear friend had passed away under not unsuspicious circumstances. The friend was in Mexico, and could not speak Spanish well, and was helping underprivileged people and homeless people, and might have been the victim of foul play, and Tom concluded that he missed him very much, and then broke off, unable to say more.

Turning to the subject of how he had been doing with the Qi Gong sessions, Tom said that as well as helping him with the physical pain he was experiencing, "It felt like it was making me feel quite a few years younger. I decreased my use of opioids to half of what I had been taking before. I didn't need to use a cane so much."

"It wasn't something that numbs you out," he added. "It was unusual. It wasn't like an opioid. It made you feel kinda like before you had those problems. It was great…"

CHAPTER ONE HUNDRED FIFTY-ONE

Subject: Qi Gong in the Treatment of Chronic Pain & Opioid Dependence - Training 4
Date: Wednesday, August 17, 2022 Minute 20

"I don't practice as much as I would like to," he said.

I inquired about the difference in the benefit he received from the medical Qi Gong compared to the self-practice Qi Gong?

"I think the practitioner-medical Qi Gong is far more effective," he responded. "I tried the self-practice a little bit - and I haven't done it as much as I would like to - but it doesn't benefit the pain as much, I don't think. The sessions with you and the other people were the ones where I really went back to feeling like where I was before I had the problems."

I asked Tom if he had a choice of doing a group self-practice with Bill and I, and a medical Qi Gong healing performed by Bill and I, which he would choose?

"I would take you and Bill doing the medical Qi Gong," he responded…

CHAPTER ONE HUNDRED FIFTY-TWO

Subject: Qi Gong in the Treatment of Chronic Pain & Opioid Dependence - Training 4
Date: Wednesday, August 17, 2022 Minute 24

Per Tom's request, Bill and I went about initiating a Qi Gong treatment: I scanned Tom first, and found there was significant energy over Tom's head that was relatively subtle and further away from Tom (in the ether level), so to suggest psychic trauma, then invited Bill to do the same. Bill also found significant energy over Tom's head.

When I inquired with Bill how he would like to approach treating Tom energetically, he responded, "I would work backwards from an onion - From the inside out."

Here I was in agreement, as this went along with my general approach to attend more definite energetics disturbances that existed in the Energy fields closer to the body, and leader attend those that were in the outer layers of the human energy field, which I would typically referred to as the Ether layer.

Before we began, Tom indicated that he had had several falls affecting his head.

"With a couple of bumps over here," he said indicating his forehead.

I invited Bill to attempt to reconcile and release the energy coming from Tom; in the process, Bill was surprised to find that more than energy coming from Tom's head, there was also a perception of energy collected on the left side of Tom a couple of feet away?

"I find it very interesting, because these two seem to match each other," he said, alluding to the energy at the top of Tom's head and that left-sided energy that was some two feet from Tom.

I determined to attempt to 'dive in' and reconcile that left-sided energy. It was literally my intention to immerse myself in this energy stream, so to 'swim in the riptide' of energy, as I challenging myself by swimming in a current of energy in attempting to reconcile difficult energy flow disturbances like this a source of enjoyment. However, Tom's energetic circulation had other ideas, as it essentially leapt right at and into my head about as soon as I began to interact with it!

This was a phenomenon that I've discussed before and refer to as 'energy transference'; that is, the movement from the participant to the practitioner, so to strongly merge with me.

I shared with Bill that this can be a surprising phenomenon for beginners, and one that might frighten a beginner, because (with the energy coming right at you and in your direction) it can feel like the energy is attacking you; however, in my experience it is nothing to be afraid of, as only good things have come out of this energetic 'merging' for both the healer and healee.

Of note, this had been the most sudden experience of energy transference that I had ever encountered. In previous energy transference experiences, I felt like, if I wanted to, I could deliberately avoid and prevent the energy from merging with me; in this case, it happened so quick and suddenly that I had no such opportunity to get out of its way or step aside and direct it elsewhere. As to why it would have been this way this time, I am not sure? Perhaps it is because I have no fear of energy transference anymore and it is responding to that greater degree of receptivity on my part? Or else it was perhaps based on the need of the Veteran to receive assistance this way?…

CHAPTER ONE HUNDRED FIFTY-THREE

Subject: Qi Gong in the Treatment of Chronic Pain & Opioid Dependence - Training 4
Date: Wednesday, August 17, 2022 Minute 32

Although still immersed in a feeling of energy of this energy transference with Tom, I took a few steps to the side, so to invite Bill to go back and scan Tom to see if he detected any energetic changes?

Bill confirmed that the energy that he had been perceiving on the left side of Tom was gone, and commented that the energy of Tom's head was moving upwards "where it needs to go and needs to keep moving."

"It's interesting, because it's a different direction," he continued. "But nonetheless that's where it wants to go."

Of note, the following day, Bill would send me a text in which he would remark of this experience as follows: "Thank you for inviting me over for Qi Gong yesterday. I wanted to mention I think you did more good for pt than I did. The upward flow of Qi was remarkable to me."

As the Qi Gong therapy session with Tom concluded, I inquired with Bill about how it is that he seems to determine when a patient has had enough based on energy flow?

"It feels like it's got an uninterrupted flow," he responded. "Like it's moving and working like a clock - All the wheels and gears are working right."

Hence, when he perceived that the impedances in flow were gone was when he determined that he had done enough.

"I do feel that 'shell effect', though," he acknowledged. "I have felt that. Like when it says, 'You have worked enough. Accept what's been done.'"

I asked Bill how often he experience the shell effect compared to that feeling of energy flow? He indicated that it was about equal between the two.

"Sometimes I feel the flow and I feel the clockwork," he said. "And sometimes it's the shell effect and like 'Hands off.'"

I inquired with Tom how he was doing?

"I'm feeling fine," he responded. "I feel very relaxed. My head feels a little ''cleaner' for the lack of a better word, and I feel good."

As for this comment of his head feeling "cleaner", it reminded me of my initial experiences in Qi Gong in which after the self-practice I would feel this "clear sensorium", whereby all of the 'buzzing' in my head was gone.

It happened that I was also feeling exceedingly good: I was feeling energy at my crown chakra and my hands beaming upwards, which was a source of delight for me - Like my idea of Nirvana…

CHAPTER ONE HUNDRED FIFTY-FOUR

Subject: Qi Gong in the Treatment of Chronic Pain & Opioid Dependence - Training 4
Date: Wednesday, August 17, 2022 Minute 37

The Innovation Accelerator folks had asked that I interview Tom as a Veteran in the program.

I asked Tom what problems were you experiencing prior to working with the Qi Gong team in the Innovation Accelerator project?

"I've had chronic pain for decades," he said, "due to wearing out the major joints in my body, mostly because of taking opioids and working with heavy weights. I was destroying my body. I've been dealing with that a long, long time."

"After my first Qi Gong session I felt lighter," he laughed. "Almost all the pain just went. Now I can pretty much deal with it comfortably myself. If I do something silly - pick up something heavy - it comes back. In general, I feel a lot younger, I guess. I'm 85 years old, so anything like that is a positive thing and it's different from what I expected it to be. More gentle. More peaceful."

I reiterated how he had said earlier that he had reduced his opioid use to half of what it had been prior to that Qi Gong treatment.

"Yes, and I don't have a bad reaction," he responded. "Because in the past, if I would cut down and one day I didn't take them, I'd be kicking my legs or thrashing around in bed or feeling horrible. Now if I don't take them, I have no problem. And it's really pretty amazing."

I asked if he was talking about Qi Gong somehow diminishing his withdrawal symptoms to opioids?

"Yeah," he responded. "Yeah. Before I would have withdrawal if I went a couple days without taking them. Usually it's two days. A lot of times I would cut down as much as I could, but the reaction I would have would be very, very bad, and so I would have to take them again. And now I can go days and days without taking them, just to make sure I don't go into any sequence of problems. But I haven't had any problems like that since my first session with you."

I asked if he had any theory as to why that might be?

"Well, truthfully, I have a lot of faith in you, Dr. Yanuck," he responded. "That probably has a lot to do with it.

"Also, I'm a strong believer in religious philosophy and some greater Power over and connected with all things. And somehow I think that's what Qi Gong did. It connected something that was already there and was helpful."

I asked if he had previously been involved in religious or spiritual practices along those lines?

"I used to do yoga and meditated quite a bit," he responded. "But it really started when I became attracted to a photograph on my yoga instructor's wall of a wild-haired young Indian man with stripes painted across his forehead. My yoga instructor explained that was 'Babaji of the Himalayas'… There are only about 10,000 Babajis in India. So, I asked him, 'What's the big deal?'

"After hesitating, the instructor said, 'A couple of old farmers discovered him in a cave near the source of the Ganges. He was immediately worshiped as the 1,000-year-old reincarnation of Shiva.'

"For non-Hindus, Shiva, known as the 'destroyer', is also the God who created, protects and transforms the universe.

"Three weeks later I was on a plane for India to meet this Babaji at his ashram.

"When I reached the stone steps leading to the ashram, I crawled through the opening. When I raised my eyes, Babaji was seated on the rusty lawn swing. Babaji's dark, medusa-like hair famed a smooth youthful face. His black onyx like eyes capturing all the light in the room. His aura was overwhelming.

"Then, he turned his attention to me.

"'Let the journalist come forward!' he boomed in broken English. I crawled across the floor on my elbows. 'Take notes,' he shouted. 'This journalist will tell the world what I am saying.'

"The ashram was located at a point on the Ganges where the river is shallow, about 3-feet deep. It's clear and cold and slippery, so that the footing on the rocky bottom was treacherous. For several hours every day, we would wade through the sacred river carrying stones often the size of a football. The more frail devotees would link arms, carrying smaller stones in baskets or wrapped in scarves. This ritual was considered a devotion.

"My second day at the ashram, Babaji interrupted the endless chanting and meditation and declared, 'You can chant the Holy name a million times, but unless you carry stones across the river to help farmers build small plots on the riverbank to grow food, your presence here doesn't make the least bit of difference.'"

So, Tom had a background in practices like these before Qi Gong.

I asked if he thought there was something different and special about Qi Gong that it was able to accomplish what it seemed that he was looking for?

"Doc, this might surprise you, but I believe the universe has a conscience," he said. "And somehow, I think that Qi Gong is part of that.

"What I feel is that what comes from Qi Gong has always been there. It's not something that comes from the heavens, like lightning – boom – and you have to get struck. It's always been existing. And now you're opening your consciousness to something that has already been there. And then allowing your consciousness to be opened so that that energy is shared everywhere else."

I asked if he thought he was in a place of being 'stuck' before perhaps doing Qi Gong, such that he wasn't able to have that unraveling process before?

"I was stuck," he admitted and laughed. "I was stuck with just the typical daily stuff of pain and the white noise of life. I got caught up with the day-to-day medication, and just a little bit of writing, but not as much as I would've liked, and this changed things. It just changed things."

Of note, Tom's description of "white noise of life" reminded me of what I would refer to as a feeling of "static" in my head that I noted would leave me with Qi Gong.

"I cut down on the opioids," he added. "I say, 'Is it the Qi Gong that made me feel better? Or is it being without the opioids that's making me feel better?' I can't say which one, but together they're working in a huge way..."

Would you say the Qi Gong was instrumental in that process?

"Yes," he asserted. "Yes, in the process of being able to be bigger than the opioids, and them not make a big influence on my life…"

When I inquired with Tom after the session, Tom provided the following input: "I felt great tranquility during the treatments by you and your student. However, I didn't notice any improvement in my normal osteoarthritis pains. Maybe I was too preoccupied... I broke my writers' block and returned to working on my stories. Don't know, but maybe it could be connected to Qi Gong?..."

CHAPTER ONE HUNDRED FIFTY-FIVE

What made this last session so special was that it marked the realization for what had been prophesized when this project was proposed. In my pitch for this project, I'd stated, "Qi Gong is a Chinese healing art that works to release the retained energy of trauma (Qi) and help the body recover optimal 'function' (Gong), so to effectively get the person back to that place of 'innocence', just like my patient with the problem of addiction desired…" Now, Tom had effectively told us that Qi Gong had helped him overcome the trauma to his dopaminergic nervous system, so to get beyond his opioid withdrawal symptoms. In this way, the last Qi Gong session brought the project full circle, bringing to fruition what had been theorized for the project.

Project MATCH is considered by many the definitive study about how best to serve patient with problems of addiction. It evaluated whether treatment should be uniform or assigned to patients based on specific needs and characteristics, and concluded that no single treatment approach is effective for all persons with addiction problems, and a more promising strategy involves assigning patients to alternative treatments based on specific needs and characteristics of patients.

Indeed, the Director of the National Institute on Alcohol Abuse and Alcoholism (NIAAA), George F. Koob, has put out a call for "Medications and behavioral therapies that reverse hyperkatifeia [addiction] by resetting brain stress, antistress, and emotional pain systems and returning them to homeostasis would be promising new targets for medication development." I hold that BioenerQi facilitates just this kind of 'reset.'

"The mind is a complicated thing," Bill commented. "It's not all just chemical. There's energies, spirit, whatever you want to call it in there. And I'm wondering if this energy work isn't going to help reset this?"

Dr. V (who had been watching the project unfold from the beginning) also commented about the complex way that Medical Qi Healing might have worked to improve Kino's brain function.

"There's crosstalk between multiple areas of the brain," he said. "And if you only confine Qi Gong to working at the frontal lobe or the motor cortex… Well, with Kino, I think there's a lot of neural activity happening. Because we are assessing motor movements. We are assessing the balance movements. The positioning of the body is important. For a nunchuk movement the brain has to calculate the movements for the position and what you do. If you don't know how to do it properly, he could hit himself or he can hit others. So, to do it properly, all these things are happening here. So, there is the coordination of the cerebellum, sensory cortex, prefrontal cortex, motor cortex… All these lobes are involved. That's why I think the crosstalk has to happen between all of these areas. So that everywhere there is a connection. It highlights the importance of connectivity. This is the perception I got when I watched you practicing Qi Gong.

"It's when that connectivity is broken that it leads to problems... When the connectivity between the temporal lobe cannot be interpreted by other parts of the brain, the person has hallucinations, and that makes them have the overstimulation of the amygdala, and that makes them fearful. PTSD the same thing: Smells from the old factory nerve, simple body sensations, the neurocircuitry is cut off after the brain has been damaged by an IED, and that makes them activate the PTSD symptoms… So that circular intactness is gone – the conductivity is gone – and it leads to many psychopathologies.

"That is why I think that the intactness of connectivity, of the brain being intact by connecting in all multiple lobes is so important… A healthy brain sign to me is when the brain is connected to all lobes and can interpret all the inputs you're getting; and that gives you a better mind analysis.

"Some think that for many schizophrenic patients, their brain activity is less and that's why they get their symptoms. But when you do the PET scan, the temporal lobe is highly activated! And that is the reason for the hallucinations.

"It's all about axonal connections. Think about wiring. Like an engineer. Like an electrician. The activation in one part of the brain is overactive, and that is not a healthy sign. The connection has to be equally distributed to make the brain feel better. And then it processes thoughts better."

Dr. V also pondered the influence of the "spiritual connection" I had with Kino and what difference that might have made in the improvements in neurologic function that we saw over the course of the Qi Gong project?

"I don't think if a different doctor, like your supervisor, Dr. F. were to stand in front of Kino and perform Qi Gong there would be the same brain energy connectivity that happens with Kino as happened with you," he asserted. "I think there is a difference. This is my theory."

"What I'm talking about is an energy of compassion," he declared, "that creates a different level of connectivity in Kino's brain. And I think there's a healing process that happens during that time, also. So, what you're doing might be different from someone else in my opinion. I don't think there would be that level of compassionate energy. I think it would be different from what you do.

"Because the patient knows that you are invested. You are caring. Do you understand the difference? I would say there would be a difference."

Yes, I believed this, too; that is, that each of us offers a certain 'frequency of healing' that can uniquely help a patient. This will be explored more thoroughly in the planned previously alluded to next work about Kino's experience (involving mental health nurse, Nancy) titled, *Shot of Love.*

"I think EEG can pick up these energy levels," Dr. V added. "Then we can find the difference between you and say Bill, and the waves created in the patient. Because your connection to the patient is different from a person who is not an expert. I think that compassion level of energy is different."

Then, he smiled.

"Do you see the happiness when I share these things?" he asked. "It's like making $1 million."

He laughed.

"That's all I want," he declared of exploring these ideas. "That's all I care for. I don't need anything else."

"But with Qi Gong, I think we need to make it scientific," he said. "We need to go to that level. That's why I think EEG is so important for us to look for those differences."

On sharing Dr. V's views with Bill, he was circumspect.

"He has his theories as to how it happened, and we have ours," he said. "Who knows what other theories people will come up with? But we saw it happen. And it's there on film. So, the question isn't, 'Is

this going to happen?' The question is, 'Is this the reason it happened?' Or 'Is that the reason it happened?' And when we get more and more of these experiences, I think it's going to be really good…"

So, with that, I'll conclude this rendering about how a small group of dedicated VA providers brought this most esoteric of medical sciences (Energy Medicine, what I believe is the final frontier in our understanding of human physiology) to the VA for the first time, successfully benefitting Veterans with complex medical conditions like TBI with neurologic deficits, and then chronic pain with opioid dependence.

Thank you for reading…

ABOUT THE AUTHOR

Michael Yanuck MD PhD is a physician-scientist whose groundbreaking research at the National Institutes of Health was the basis for an FDA-approved vaccine for cancer. Following a traumatic leg injury, he trained in Bioenergy and Qi Gong, introduced Energy Medicine techniques at the National Center for Complementary and Integrative Health, and worked with Chi Gong Masters who were part of the President's Executive Committee on Alternative Medicine. For his work with Veterans in the Innovation Accelerator Qi Gong project, he received the 2023 Science of Tai Chi & Qigong Award from Harvard University and has plans to continue this work at Yale University.

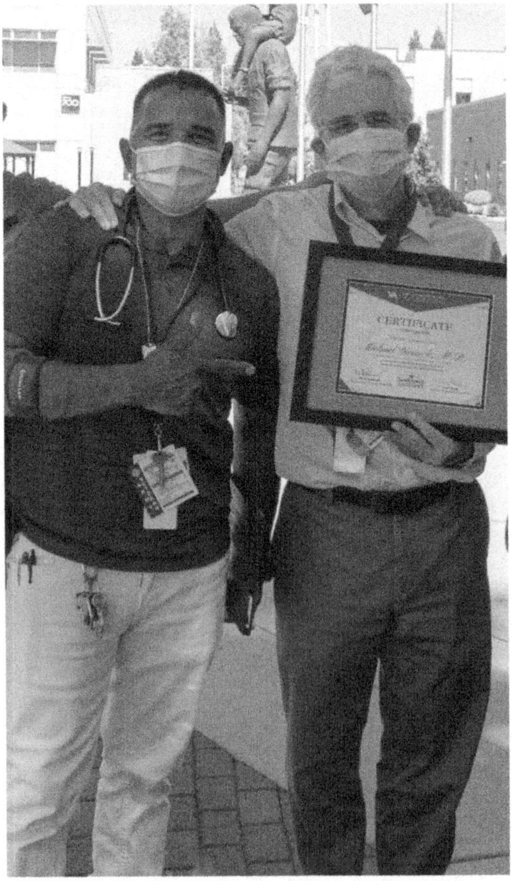

Made in the USA
Monee, IL
04 November 2026

67376423R00154